INSOMNIA

84 Sleep Hacks To Fall Asleep Fast, Sleep Better and Have Sweet Dreams Without Sleeping Pills

Disclaimer: The ideas and suggestions contained in this book are not intended as a substitute for consulting with your physician. All matters regarding your health require medical supervision.

"Some people talk in their sleep. Lecturers talk while other people sleep"

Albert Camus

"All men whilst they are awake are in one common world. But each of them, when he is asleep, is in a world of his own."

Plutarch

TABLE OF CONTENTS

PART B – HOW TO SLEEP BETTER

PART C – RECAP

1. INTRODUCTION

"You're not healthy, unless your sleep is healthy."

Dr. William Dement

Sleep is weird. Think about it: for about one-third of every day, you lie down with your eyes closed, while your system shuts down. The stage performer that sings the most beautiful song, the chef that cooks the most delicious risotto, the athlete that just ran a world record today: when they close their eyes, they are no more. Until they wake up, and do the same thing all over again.

Yet, without sufficient sleep, all the beauty in the world around us created by mankind could not exist. That eggs benedict your local dinner serves for breakfast. The elevator taking you up to the office. The office chair you are sitting in. The car you are driving. The air conditioner controlling the room temperature. The book you are reading right now…

All of this could not exist if the people involved in their creation would not be able to sleep.

Sleep really is the **cornerstone** of **life.**

But what is sleep? How does it affect your daily performance and overall health? And what can you do to sleep better if you are sleep deprived?

I am glad you asked! Because you have come to the right place. By reading this book, all these questions will be addressed and answered. And not only that, you will learn so much more!

This book consists of three parts:

1. **Part A – Sleep Explained**
2. **Part B – How To Sleep Better**
3. **Part C – Recap**

Part A – Sleep Explained: in the first part of this book, you will learn the basics of sleep. Before we get into the juicy stuff of how you can hack the quality of your sleep, it is important to get a good understanding of how sleep works. We will cover why we sleep and dream, how sleep works, how much sleep we need, and sleep disorders. By the time you have completed reading Part A you will know all the basics of sleep!

Every chapter in 'Part A – Sleep Explained' starts with the **Key Takeaway** of that chapter. This allows you to quickly get the gist of every chapter before you start reading it.

Part B – How To Sleep Better: the second part is all about strategies you can use to improve the quality of your sleep. We will debunk a number of common sleep myths, and then talk about what *does* work. How to turn your bedroom and bed into a safe and sacred space for sleep and relaxation, how exposure to light and electronics impact your sleep, and a bunch of other strategies you can use to induce sleep.

Where the first part of this book is more about learning what sleep is all about, 'Part B – How To Sleep Better' focuses on taking action. You will learn a ton of strategies you can use to fall asleep more easily and sleep more soundly. However, merely reading this book is not enough. The real magic happens when you implement the tactics and techniques included in this book. Therefore, the second part of this book is loaded with practical **Sleep Hacks**. These are action steps will put you in pole position, giving you the best possible shot at improving the quality of your sleep.

Part C – Recap: at the end of this book, you will find a recap of all the **Key Takeaways** and **Sleep Hacks**. This is an excellent resource you can always get back to if you want to review what you have learned.

Being sleep deprived can affect every part of your being. It can make you:

- feel moody
- be less productive
- be forgetful, and
- be the catalyst for a variety of diseases

But you no longer need to be a victim of insomnia!

Now is the time to **take back control** your life and learn how to **sleep like a baby** again.

Take your last yawn now.

Let's dive into it!

PART A

SLEEP EXPLAINED

2. WHAT IS SLEEP

"Sleeping is no mean art: for its sake one must stay awake all day."

Friedrich Nietzsche

Key Takeaway: *Sleep is a natural and recurring period of rest for the mind and body. During sleep, you are not conscious, you are mostly immobile, and your sensitivity to external stimuli is diminished.*

2.1 Introduction

Zzzzzzz....

We go to sleep every night. At some point in the late evening we call it a day, and prepare ourselves for the night. We close the curtains, undress, brush our teeth, turn off the lights. We roll in bed and cover ourselves with a blanket to keep ourselves warm. Some people fall asleep almost immediately. For some others it may take a bit longer. But for the average American it takes no more than twenty-two minutes to fall asleep, according to 2008 research by the Centers for Disease Control and Prevention (goo.gl/LxZWC2). And after a good night sleep, we wake up in the morning and start a new day, hopefully rested and recharged!

Unfortunately, falling asleep isn't that easy for everyone. Chances are that you picked up this book because you have trouble falling asleep, or even suffer from a sleep disorder. We will get into that later on.

***

2.2 Sleep Definitions

But what is sleep?

Let's look at a few definitions, and see what elements they all have in common. The key elements in each definition are in bold.

For its article on 'Sleep', Wikipedia quotes the definition in the Macmillan Dictionary for Students:

*"Sleep is a **naturally recurring state** characterized by **reduced or absent consciousness**, relatively **suspended sensory activity**, and **inactivity** of nearly all **voluntary muscles**".*

The Oxford English Dictionary defines sleep as:

*"A condition of body and mind which typically **recurs** for several hours every night, in which the **nervous system is inactive**, the eyes closed, the **postural muscles relaxed**, and **consciousness** practically **suspended**".*

According to the Dorland's Medical Dictionary for Health Consumers, sleep is:

*"A period of **rest for the body and mind**, during which **volition** and **consciousness** are in **abeyance** and **bodily functions** are **partially suspended**; also described as a behavioral state, with characteristic **immobile posture** and **diminished** but readily reversible **sensitivity to external stimuli**."*

And finally, the American Heritage® Medical Dictionary defines sleep as:

*"A **natural periodic state** of **rest for the mind and body**, in which the **eyes usually close** and **consciousness** is completely or partially **lost**, so that there is a **decrease in bodily movement** and **responsiveness to external stimuli**. During sleep the brain undergoes a characteristic cycle of brain-wave activity that includes intervals of dreaming."*

***

2.3 Common Elements In These Sleep Definitions

Some of these definitions are a bit technical. But when we examine them closely, we can see that most of them have the following in common.

Sleep is:

- a period of rest for the mind and body
- natural
- recurring
- a state in which we are not conscious
- a state in which our voluntary muscles are relaxed, and we are mostly immobile
- a state in which our sensitivity to external stimuli is diminished

This is what happens to you every night. And although you can be deeply, very deeply asleep, rest assured that sleep is much easier to reverse than a state of hibernation or coma. It is a matter of hours before you wake up, not weeks or even longer!

Now that you know what sleep is, let's take a closer look at why we sleep.

3. WHY DO WE SLEEP

"It is a common experience that a problem difficult at night is resolved in the morning after the committee of sleep has worked on it."

John Steinbeck

Key Takeaway: *There is no definitive answer as to why we sleep. What we do know is that sleep helps conserve energy, repair and rejuvenate the body, and develop the brain. There are many health benefits to getting enough sleep, whereas being sleep deprived can put you at risk for heart disease or a stroke, lower sex drive, and affect your mood.*

3.1 Introduction

Wouldn't it be great if we didn't have to sleep at all? Imagine how much more we could achieve if only we would be able to use all twenty-four hours in a day!

Unfortunately, it doesn't work that way. After being awake for a while, inevitably you get tired and will want to go to sleep.

We spent roughly one-third of our lives sleeping. But with the exception of the occasional dream memory, most of us have no idea what happens when we close our eyes.

3.2 Why Do We Sleep

So why do we sleep? This is a question that is surprisingly difficult to answer.

There are a number of theories that take a shot at trying to explain why we sleep:

- **Energy conservation**: this theory suggests that we sleep to conserve energy. Our metabolism is significantly reduced during sleep. The brain constitutes about 3% of your body weight, but it uses 20-25% of your body's energy! So reducing metabolism would increase our chances of survival.
- **Restoration**: this theory suggests that we sleep to repair and rejuvenate our body. Recent scientific research has shown for example that major restorative functions in the body mostly occur when we sleep, like the release of growth hormones, or muscle growth.
- **Brain development**: this theory suggests that we sleep to develop our brain. For example, sleep plays an important role in the brain development of children. And as we will see below, when adults are sleep deprived, their ability to learn and adequately perform their tasks is impaired.

But as things stand today, these are only theories. When asked about the reason why we sleep, William Dement, a sleep researcher and founder of the Sleep Research Center at Stanford

University, said: *"As far as I know, the only reason we need to sleep that is really, really solid is because we get sleepy."*

In one of the most famous scientific research experiments conducted with regard to finding out why we sleep, the sleep researcher Allan Rechtschaffen deprived rats of sleep until they died. He would, probably much to the dismay of animal rights activists, place a rat on a disk suspended on a spindle over a tank of water. Whenever the rat fell asleep, the disk would turn and the rat would fall in the water. This would wake the rat up immediately. Not surprisingly, all the rats were dead after about two weeks.

After the rats had died, Rechtschaffen performed necropsies on them. He wanted to see if there were any physiological changes in the rats as a consequence of the sleep deprivation. However, their organs were not damaged. He didn't find anything wrong with them. So it appeared that they had indeed died simply from sleep deprivation.

***

3.3 Negative Side Effects Of Sleep Deprivation

So far, researchers have not been able to pinpoint yet exactly why we need sleep. We do know however that if we don't sleep, or don't sleep enough, there are negative side effects.

A number of major disasters were caused by a lack of sleep. Perhaps most well known is the explosion of the Chernobyl power plant in 1986, described by some as the worst nuclear disaster in world history. The power plant exploded after the engineers involved had been working for thirteen hours or more.

Another disaster that was found to be related to lack of sleep is the explosion of the Challenger Space Shuttle, also in 1986. In a report (goo.gl/p1Reiw) investigating the events preceding the fatal explosion, it was found that:

"Certain key managers had obtained <2 h sleep the night before and had been on duty since 1:00 a.m. that morning.

It was further found that:

"time pressure, particularly that caused by launch scrubs and turnarounds, increased the potential for sleep loss and judgment errors",

and that working

"excessive hours, while admirable, raises serious questions when it jeopardizes job performance, particularly when critical management decisions are at stake"

There is a long list of negative side effects associated with sleep deprivation. For example, sleep deprivation:

- can cause health problems, like putting you at risk for heart disease, high blood pressure or a stroke
- lowers sex drive
- affects our mood, and can even result in depression

- can reduce our ability to learn efficiently, because it impairs attention, alertness, and concentration
- can impair our ability to make sound judgments

***

3.4 The Benefits Of Getting Enough Sleep

On the flipside, getting enough sleep is associated with a wide number of benefits. Not surprisingly, some of these are the opposite of the negative side effects we just covered.

Getting enough sleep:

- improves your health
- increases sex drive
- improves your mood
- makes you think clearer
- improves your memory

This is something anyone can attest to. Science may not have figured out why it is exactly that we sleep. But you and I both know that we feel better when we get enough sleep, and feel worse when we are sleep deprived.

4. HOW DOES SLEEP WORK

"I love sleep. My life has a tendency to fall apart when I'm awake, you know?"

Ernest Hemingway

<u>Key Takeaway</u>: *Sleep proceeds in 90-minute cycles of NREM and REM sleep. These are not identical: as the night progresses, we spend more time in REM sleep in later sleep cycles. Moreover, the amount of NREM and REM sleep is influenced by the time of day.*

4.1 Introduction

So far, we've covered what sleep is, and why we sleep. Next, we'll discuss how sleep actually works.

***

4.2 Types Of Sleep

Sleep occurs in periods of approximately ninety minutes. There are two types of sleep:

1. Non-Rapid-Eye-Movement (NREM) sleep
2. Rapid-Eye-Movement (REM) sleep

NREM and REM sleep are very different. In fact, they differ so much that physiologists even classify them as distinct behavioral states.

***

4.3 NREM Sleep

NREM sleep may be best defined as any sleep that is not REM Sleep. That may sound a bit vague right now, but it will make more sense after you have read about REM sleep below. NREM sleep is basically the dreamless part of the sleep cycle. Everything slows down: your breathing, heart rate, blood pressure, and body movement.

NREM sleep consists of 3 stages:

1. **N1 (5 - 10% of total sleep in adults; 1 to 7 minutes per cycle)**: this is a stage of light sleep that usually occurs between sleep and wakefulness, and can also sometimes occur between periods of deeper sleep and periods of REM. In this stage you can be awakened easily. The eyes still move slowly. And quite a few people experience sudden muscle contractions during this stage.
2. **N2 (45 - 55% of total sleep in adults; 10 to 25 minutes per cycle)**: in this stage, eye movement stops. Also, brain waves become slower. Muscle activity decreases, and conscious awareness of the external environment fades completely.

3. **N3 (15 - 25% of total sleep in adults; 20 to 40 minutes per cycle)**: this stage is referred to as deep sleep, or also as slow-wave or delta sleep. There is no eye movement, and also no muscle activity. It is very difficult to wake someone from this sleep stage. The sleeper is no longer aware of any external stimuli, and is more or less cut off from the outside world.

There used to be a fourth stage, N4. However, the American Academy of Sleep Medicine stage has merged N4 with N3 in their 2007 manual for the scoring of sleep and associated events.

***

4.4 REM Sleep

REM sleep is the most well known of the two types of sleep. It is even what the alternative rock band R.E.M., most famous for their hit 'Losing My Religion', named themselves after!

This type of sleep is characterized by random movement of the eyes. Hence the name. Among other things, REM sleep is associated with dreaming. Many sleep experts think that the rapid eye movements during REM sleep are actually in some way related to dreams.

In REM sleep, almost all the muscles in the body are temporarily paralyzed. The purpose is probably to prevent us from actually acting out what we are seeing and doing in our dreams. Which would potentially be very dangerous, both to ourselves and the ones around us!

A tragic example is that of Brian Thomas, who suffered from night terrors all his life. For this reason, him and his wife slept in separate bedrooms. However, one night, when they were on a holiday travelling, they slept in the same bed in their camper. In his sleep, he strangled his wife while dreaming that someone had broken into the camper. Later on, he was acquitted of murder charges, but for the rest of the life has to live with the guilt of knowing that his wife died at his hands.

***

4.5 How Long Do We Spend In NREM And REM Sleep

Adults spent roughly 80% in the NREM sleep and 20-25% in the REM sleep. Infants spend a lot more time in REM sleep: almost 50%. On the other hand, older adults spend progressively less time in REM sleep.

***

4.6 Sleep Cycles

Sleep proceeds in cycles of NREM and REM, and usually in this order. A sleep cycle lasts about ninety minutes, and we usually have about four or five of them per night.

The first four stages make up our NREM sleep, whereas the fifth stage is the REM sleep. A sleep cycle proceeds in the following order:

$$N1 \rightarrow N2 \rightarrow N3 \rightarrow N2 \rightarrow REM$$

The cycles are not identical, however. During the night, the amount of time spent in a particular stage starts to shift:

- In the first 2-3 sleep cycles, we spend most of our time in N3 (NREM sleep).
- But in the final 2-3 sleep cycles, we spend much more time in REM sleep, accompanied by lighter NREM sleep.

And to make matters even more complicated, the amount of NREM and REM sleep one gets is also partly determined by the time of day. In general, one experiences:

- more NREM sleep earlier in the night
- more REM sleep later in the night

This means that if you were to go to bed late, you would probably get more REM sleep compared to someone who goes to bed early.

But what makes you want to go to sleep and wake up in the first place? That is what we will cover next.

5. HOW LIGHT AFFECTS YOUR SLEEP

"The worst thing in the world is to try to sleep and not to."

F. Scott Fitzgerald

__Key Takeaway__: Your circadian rhythm is a body clock that controls when you are alert and sleepy. It is not only influenced by natural factors, but also by external factors such as light, time and melatonin. To improve your sleep quality, make sure you see lots of natural (sun)light during the day, and reduce your light exposure in the evening.

5.1 Introduction

The time at which you start feeling drowsy, and the time at which you start waking up, are both governed by your circadian rhythm. The circadian rhythm is basically a twenty-four hour clock governing when you are alert and when you are asleep. It is also known as the sleep/wake cycle.

The circadian rhythm is partly produced by natural factors within the body, but it is also impacted by external factors such as light, time and melatonin.

***

5.2 The Connection Between Light and Melatonin

Melatonin is a hormone secreted by the pineal gland. It regulates when we feel sleepy and when we feel alert. It is heavily affected by the body's exposure to light. When it is dark, the pineal gland secretes more melatonin, and when it is light, it is secreted less. By releasing more melatonin when it is dark, our body receives the signal to prepare for sleep, and we become more drowsy. The opposite effect happens when melatonin secretion is reduced. This is a system that has been shaped and fine-tuned over many years of evolution, adapting to the sun coming up and going down.

Yet, with our modern lifestyles we can really mess up how much melatonin is secreted, and consequently screw up our circadian rhythm. Often, we work in offices where our exposure to light is less than if we were to spend the day being outside. Also, with the sun coming up later in wintertime, many of us wake up and leave the house when it is still dark.

Conversely, in the evening, when it is already dark outside, we are exposed to light not just from the lighting in our house, but also to the blue light emitted by all the electronic devices around the house: our television, laptop, phone.

If you are looking to fall asleep more easily and sleep more soundly, make sure you see lots of natural (sun)light during the day, and reduce your light exposure in the evening. Many of the sleep improvement strategies laid out later on this book are based on this key takeaway.

So now you know the basics of how sleep works. But how much sleep do you actually need?

6. HOW MUCH SLEEP DO WE NEED

"One of the Georges - I forget which - once said that a certain number of hours' sleep each night - I cannot recall at the moment how many - made a man something which for the time being has slipped my memory."

P.G. Wodehouse, Something Fresh

*<u>**Key Takeaway**</u>: Most people need around 7-8 hours of sleep. Short sleepers can be categorized in two types: natural and habitual short sleepers. Natural short sleepers are rare, but due to a gene mutation they reap the benefits of a full night of sleep in nearly half the time. Habitual short sleepers on the other hand have trained themselves to sleep less. However, they take a risk, as they are not immune to the long-term risks of keeping themselves awake.*

6.1 Introduction

In his book 'Think Like a Billionaire', Donald Trump wrote: *"Don't sleep any more than you have to, I usually sleep about four hours per night."* And when he was at an event in Springfield, Illinois campaigning for the 2016 elections, he said: *"You know, I'm not a big sleeper. I like three hours, four hours, I toss, I turn, I beep-de-beep, I want to find out what's going on."*

And Trump is not the only one with this sleep habit. Other people that have been reported to sleep as little as four hours a night are:

- **Thomas Edison**, producer of the first commercially viable light bulb, and inventor of the phonograph
- **Martha Stewart**, business woman, founder of Living Omnimedia and award-winning television show host, entrepreneur and bestselling author
- **Indra Nooyi**, Chairperson and Chief Executive Officer of PepsiCo

And in his book 'The 4 Hour Body', Tim Ferriss writes about sleeping less by using what is called the Uberman Sleep Schedule. This is a polyphasic sleep schedule consisting entirely of 20-minute naps, for a total of just three hours in six portions distributed equally throughout the day.

The implicit message of the likes of Donald Trump and Martha Stewart is that success can only be achieved by giving up hours of sleep. So is everyone who sleeps more than that just lazy?

The simple answer is: No.

***

6.2 The Average Adult Needs Seven Or More Hours Of Sleep Per Night

There may be a small percentage of people that are naturally short sleepers. But most people need around eight hours of sleep. In fact, in a June 2015 Sleep Journal publication, the American Academy of Sleep Medicine (AASM) and the Sleep Research Society both recommend at least seven or more hours of sleep per night for adults aged 18 to 60 years, to avoid the health risks of chronic inadequate sleep (goo.gl/yFR7lw).

When commenting on this publication, Dr. Nathaniel F. Watson of AASM said:

"Sleep is critical to health, along with a healthy diet and regular exercise. Our Consensus Panel found that sleeping six or fewer hours per night is inadequate to sustain health and safety in adults, and agreed that seven or more hours of sleep per night is recommended for all healthy adults."

***

6.3 But What About Short Sleepers?

Short sleepers can be categorized in two types:

- natural short sleepers
- habitual short sleepers

***

6.4 Natural Short Sleepers

Natural short sleepers are rare, but they do exist. They carry a mutation of the so-called DEC2 gene. The first scientist to publish about this was Ying-Hui Fu, a geneticist at the University of California at San Francisco. In a 2009 Science article (goo.gl/p8gi1P), she reports finding a mother-daughter pair who could both get away with only six hours of sleep. Without any ill effects. After examining their genes and comparing it to other test subjects, Fu found that both mother and daughter had the same mutation of the DEC2 gene.

So basically, natural short sleepers reap the benefits of a full night of sleep in nearly half the time.

***

6.5 Habitual Short Sleepers

Habitual short sleepers on the other hand are those that have trained themselves to sleep less. There are many different ways of training yourself to sleep less than seven to eight hours per night. From just getting out of bed every morning at 5 a.m., to following the Uberman Sleep Schedule. It takes some time for the body to develop and adapt to the new habit of short-term sleep. For example, when following the Uberman Sleep Schedule, people report feeling like a zombie for the first three to four weeks. But after a while they will be able to conquer the short-term effects of being sleep deprived, like lack of focus, bad mood, et cetera.

However, habitual short sleepers take a risk. Although they may attain short-term benefits, such as increased productivity, they are in danger of suffering long-term health consequences. They do not have the DEC2 gene mutation and are therefore not immune to the long-term risks of keeping themselves awake. The brain needs a full seven to eight hours of sleep every night in order to flush out chemicals it doesn't need, and to recharge. By not allowing this process to complete, habitual short sleepers put themselves at increased risk for a number of diseases, such as Alzheimer.

***

6.6 Get Enough Sleep

So are Donald Trump or Martha Stewart natural or habitual short sleepers? Who knows...

But for most of us it is safe to assume that we are not natural short sleepers. And while there are definitely short-term benefits to establishing a short sleep habit, you may put your long-term health at risk.

And to give you a final push, here is what Arianna Huffington wrote about getting enough sleep in her book 'Thrive':

"We think, mistakenly, that success is the result of the amount of time we put in at work, instead of the quality of time we put in. Sleep, or how little of it we need, has become a symbol of our prowess. We make a fetish of not getting enough sleep, and we boast about how little sleep we get. I once had dinner

with a man who bragged to me that he'd gotten only four hours of sleep the night before. I resisted the temptation to tell him that the dinner would have been a lot more interesting if he had gotten five."

So listen to your body, and make sure to get seven or more hours of sleep per night.

7. WHY DO WE DREAM

"The best thing about dreams is that fleeting moment, when you are between asleep and awake, when you don't know the difference between reality and fantasy, when for just that one moment you feel with your entire soul that the dream is reality, and it really happened."

James Arthur Baldwin

Key Takeaway: *Dreams have fascinated mankind for thousands of years. We now know that dreams mainly occur in REM sleep, are necessary, and being deprived of REM sleep causes all kinds of behavioral changes. Different theories suggest that dreams help us form memories, help our brain to process challenging experiences and emotions, and helps us with our survival. But these are only theories: why we dream still remains very much a mystery.*

7.1 Introduction

Friedrich August Kekulé, a 19th century German organic chemist, was one of the most prominent chemists in Europe. He was the principal founder of the theory of chemical structure, and his most famous work was on the structure of benzene.

When speaking at the 25th anniversary of the benzene structure discovery in 1890, Kekulé explained how the theory came about: in a dream.

After another day of unsuccessfully trying to solve the problem of the benzene structure, he dozed off in his chair next to his fireplace. Then he had dream. In it, he saw atoms dancing around, and linking to one another. Later, he had another dream. Again he saw atoms dance around. However, this time the atoms also formed themselves into strings, ultimately arranging into the form of a snake. That image then evolved into a snake biting its own tail.

It was this dream that made Kekulé realize that benzene molecules are made up of rings of carbon atoms.

**

7.2 Inspirational Dreams

There are many other stories of people inventing or creating new things after a dream:

- James Cameron came up with the idea for the film 'The Terminator' in a fever dream. He dreamt of a robot coming out of an explosion, cut in half, armed with kitchen knives, crawling toward a fleeing girl. After he woke up, Cameron made a sketch of the robot. And not much later he started writing the script for 'The Terminator'.

- Einstein discovered the foundation of the principle of relativity in a dream. When he was young, he dreamed he was hurtling down a mountainside. As he went faster and faster, he approached the speed of light. When he looked at this point, he noticed that stars were altered in appearance in relation to him. This dream led him to discover that E=mc2.
- Paul McCartney composed the melody of 'Yesterday' in a dream. After he woke up, he immediately ran to the piano to write it down. In 1980, McCartney explained: *"I liked the melody a lot, but because I'd dreamed it I couldn't believe I'd written it. I thought, 'No, I've never written like this before.' But I had the tune, which was the most magic thing."*

How about that, huh?

Most people however never have these kinds of dreams. They just dream about sitting in purple grass hanging out with their friend James, who suddenly morphs into Britney Spears, as T-Rex hammers fly through the sky. And the dreamer doesn't even blink…

And then there are those that say they don't dream at all.

But why do we dream?

***

7.3 A Brief History Of Dream Research

Dreams have always fascinated mankind. For thousands of years, people have wondered what the function of dreaming is, and if dreams have meaning. Different theories on why we dream have been developed, which we will get to in a minute.

What really changed the game though was the discovery in 1953 of REM sleep, by Nathaniel Kleitman, PhD, chair of physiology at the University of Chicago. Before, it was believed that there was just one sleep state. But when studying sleep disorders in infants, Dr. Kleitman had noticed that sometimes the eyes would move very rapidly. Later on, he and his team found that adults showed the same behavior. Wanting to explore what this might mean, the researchers woke up the subjects during the REM sleep. Most of the time, the subjects reported that they were dreaming. Conversely, when they were woken up during NREM sleep, dreams were rarely reported. This was a major breakthrough.

Then, in 1960, William Dement started studying the effects of REM sleep deprivation. If you recall, Dement is the sleep researcher quoted in the chapter 'Why Do Sleep' saying: *"As far as I know, the only reason we need to sleep that is really, really solid is because we get sleepy."* He and his team decided to wake up subjects just after the onset of dreaming and to continue this procedure throughout the night. Not just to check if they were indeed dreaming. But also to observe how being woken up in REM sleep would affect the subjects.

To make sure that any findings couldn't simply be accounted to the multiple awakenings, they also used a control group who would be subjected to an identical routine. However, instead of waking them up during REM sleep, these subjects would be woken up during NREM sleep.

The result?

- The subjects that were woken up during REM sleep experienced psychological disturbances such as anxiety, irritability, and difficulty in concentrating
- One person even quit the study in an apparent panic
- Two other subjects found the test was too stressful and they stopped one night short of the goal of five nights of dream deprivation
- At least one subject exhibited serious anxiety and agitation
- Five subjects developed an increase in appetite, and three subjects actually gained 3 - 5 pounds during the test

And perhaps most importantly: NONE of these changes were seen in the NREM sleep control group!

This led Dement to conclude *"that a certain amount of dreaming each night is a necessity. (...) It is possible that if the dream suppression were carried on long enough, a serious disruption of the personality would result."*

***

7.4 Why Do We Dream?

We now know that:

- Dreams mainly occur in REM sleep
- Dreaming is necessary
- Being deprived of REM sleep causes all kinds of behavioral changes

So science has made great progress in deepening our understanding of dreams. But that doesn't explain why we dream.

Unfortunately, the role of dreaming is still very much a mystery. Views on what dreams might mean have varied and changed through time and culture.

In ancient times, kings would have advisers at their court to interpret dreams and explain mysteries. For example, the Bible (Daniel 2) contains the story of the Babylonian king Nebuchadnezzar having a troubling dream. Instead of asking his astrologers to explain its meaning, he told them to first also tell him what he had dreamed. After all, they were communicating with the Gods, weren't they? If they failed, they would be executed. Ultimately, Daniel saved the day after the dream and its meaning had been revealed to him in a vision.

Different cultures, like the Greek and the Roman, believed that dreams were direct messages from God or deceased persons, predicting the future. Similar beliefs can be found in Mayan and Native Indian culture.

The psychological theory that has been predominant since the 20th century is that dreams reveal insight into hidden desires and emotions. This theory was developed by Sigmund Freud, most known for his work in the field of psychoanalysis. In this view, dreams are a reflection of desires and anxieties stored deep within us, possibly going back to repressed childhood memories or obsessions.

Carl Jung expanded on that, and pointed out dreams convey messages that we can use to uncover and help resolve certain problems and fears that we may have. This is especially true for recurring dreams. According to Jung, if a dream is recurring, this means that the dreamer is neglecting a part of their life related to the dream.

I can personally attest to that. Many years ago, when I was working seventy to eighty hours a week in a corporate job, I would have this recurring dream. I would find myself in my house. Each time the house would look different, it was never the actual house I lived in at the time. But it was clear that this was my house. And what would happen is that I would find a secret room. So my house was actually much bigger than I originally thought! From what I remember, most of the times that new room was still empty. But just knowing that I had this extra room gave me a feeling of spaciousness, and also excitement! All the things I could do with that room…

At one point in my career I made the choice to quit my job, and travel to South-East Asia. Originally I planned to travel for a year, and find myself a job again back home. However, over time, my life slowly evolved into one where I now work location independently. And ever since I left my corporate job, I never had this recurring dream again.

Nowadays, besides psychology, there are also theories from different scientific disciplines such as psychiatry and neuro-biology, trying to explain why we dream. These include:

- **Dreams helps up form memories**: Learning new information happens in three phases: acquisition, consolidation, and recall. According to scientific research, our memories are formed and consolidated through the strengthening of the neural connections during sleep.
- **Dreams help our brain to process complicated, challenging and upsetting experiences and emotions that took place when we were awake**: The purpose is to achieve and maintain emotional and psychological balance.
- **Dreams helps us with our survival**: By working through unsettling experiences and feelings at night, our brain prepares us to deal with future challenges, threats and dangers in the best possible way.
- **Dreams are the result of our brain simply firing away**: When we go to sleep, everything slows down. We don't need to concentrate like we do during the daytime. There are no survival consequences if we make a mistake. As a result, our brain gets a free pass and makes very loose connections. This has even led some to propose that dreams have no purpose at all.

There is probably never going to be one single theory that will give us the definitive answer as to why we dream. If we will ever be able to fully explain why we dream, it is likely that dreaming is found to serve multiple functions.

An interesting analogy that might help visualize this, is the popular 'God is an elephant' analogy, used to show that all religions are valid ways to describe God. In this analogy, there are four blind men who discover an elephant. They have obviously never seen an elephant. As a matter of fact, they have never even heard of an elephant. Let alone touched one. So they approach the elephant, one at a time, placing their hands on it, feeling it. And then they try to describe the elephant to their fellow blind friends. The first one touches the elephant's side and announces it is a like a wall. The second one gets a hold of the elephant's leg, and concludes it is a like a tree. Another finds the trunk, and says: *"You are both wrong: it is like a snake"*. And finally, the last blind man grabs a hold of the elephant's tail and concludes that it is like a rope.

All of them are partly right, yet none of them see the full picture! It is the same with the dream theories. These different theories may all partly explain why we dream. And yet there is still so much we don't know about why we dream...

8. WHAT ARE SLEEP DIS- ORDERS

"With insomnia, nothing's real. Everything's far away. Every- thing's a copy of a copy of a copy. When you have insomnia, you are never really asleep, and you are never really awake."

Edward Norton in the movie 'Fight Club'

<u>Key Takeaway</u>: Being sleep deprived can have a detrimental impact on your life. Sleep disorders come in different forms, and the cause can vary depending on the type and severity of the sleep disorder, as well as the individual. Sleep disorders are treated with either medical treatment or psychotherapeu- tic/behavioral treatment. For the first, consult your physician. The second part of this book contains behavioral strategies you can use to tackle sleep deprivation and improve the quali- ty of your sleep.

8.1 Introduction

Many people have trouble falling asleep, or staying asleep after they finally dozed off.

Some well-known people that suffered from sleeplessness are Napoleon Bonaparte, Abraham Lincoln, Marilyn Monroe, and Vincent van Gogh. Van Gogh wrote about his insomnia many times in letters addressed to his brother Theo, for example in September 1884:

"I cannot eat, and I cannot sleep - that is to say, not enough, and that makes one weak."

Sleep deprivation can have a detrimental impact on our lives. Some of the negative effects of not getting enough sleep are:

- Difficult to concentrate
- Depression
- Getting angered easily
- Hallucination
- Weakened immune response
- Increased risk of Type 2 Diabetes

Basically, everything we feel, experience and want to do during the day becomes more difficult if we cannot sleep during the night.

***

8.2 Types Of Sleep Disorders

Sleep disorders come in different forms, and are often classified in groups describing how they affect you or why they happen.

Some of the most common types of sleep disorders are:

- **Insomnia**: it is difficult to fall and stay asleep

- **Sleep Apnea**: the airway is obstructed while being asleep. People with this sleep disorder often snore, and experience a lack of enough deep sleep
- **Restless Legs Syndrome (RLS)**: a sleep movement disorder, causing an irresistible urge to move the legs while trying to fall asleep
- **Narcolepsy**: people with this condition experience extreme daytime sleepiness. They can also often fall asleep spontaneously at any time.

And this is by no means an exhaustive list. There are many more sleep disorders. These are just some of the disorders that are diagnosed most often.

***

8.3 What Causes Sleep Disorders?

The cause of a sleep disorder depends on the type and severity of the sleep disorder, and furthermore very much on the individual.

There are a variety of possible causes for a sleep disorder, such as:

- **Stress**, for example caused by a break-up, or losing your dog
- **Physical discomforts**, like pain from an injury, or sunburn
- **Medical issues**, like asthma

- **Mental disorders**, such as anxiety disorders or depression
- **Diet**, like drinking a lot of alcohol, or coffee
- **Environment**, like moving to a busy city center and not (yet) adapting to the noise pollution, or a heat wave
- **Aging**. As we will see in chapter 9 'Seven Sleep Myths Debunked', older people sleep less because of the discomforts that come with aging.
- **Genetics**. For example, there is scientific research suggesting that there is a genetic basis for narcolepsy.
- **Medication**, like blood pressure medication, or antidepressants

***

8.4 Treatment Of Sleep Disorders

With so many sleep disorders, and so many potential causes, there is not a single way of treating them.

Generally speaking, sleep disorders are treated with:

- Medical treatment
- Psychotherapeutic or behavioral treatment

Which one is the best fit for a particular sleep disorder needs to be decided on a case-by-case basis. The correct diagnosis and suggested treatment does not only take into account the particular sleep disorder, but also the patient's medical and psychiatric history, as well as his lifestyle habits. The best results can often be gained by setting up a program that contains elements from different types of treatment, tailored to the patient and her sleep disorder.

***

8.5 Medical Treatment

The most popular medical treatment are sleeping pills. However, although they may temporarily alleviate the sleep disorder symptoms, they do not treat the cause. Therefore, sleeping pills are not a long-term solution. Moreover, sleeping pills come with significant side effects, such as:

- Headache
- Constipation or diarrhea
- Feeling weak
- Daytime drowsiness
- Heartburn
- Difficulty keeping balance
- Stomach pain

And finally, you can quickly build up tolerance when you take sleeping pills daily over a long period of time. This means needing higher prescribed doses to get the same effect. And that is something you should avoid, given the many side effects that sleeping pills can have.

Other medical treatments are taking supplements, treating underlying health problems, surgery (for apnea), or wearing a mouthpiece or even a sleep apnea mask at night.

***

8.6 Psychotherapeutic Or Behavioral Treatment

An alternative for medical treatment, especially as a first resort, is psychotherapeutic or behavioral treatment, better known as cognitive behavioral therapy. This type of treatment is especially used to treat insomnia.

Cognitive behavioral therapy aims to tackle patterns of thinking or behavior that may cause the sleep disorder. This is done by trying to identify those thoughts and behaviors, and replacing them with habits that promote good sleep. Cognitive behavioral therapy deals with the root of the sleep disorder and tries to eradicate it, whereas sleeping pills only treat the symptoms.

***

8.7 What's Ahead

The purpose of this book is to help you understand the importance of sleep, and to help you improve the quality and duration of your sleep.

The use of medical treatment for sleep disorders is outside the scope of this book. First off, in many cases medication often only treats the symptoms and does not offer a long-term solution. Moreover, I am not a doctor. If you would like to know more about possible medical treatments for a sleep disorder you may be suffering from, I recommend you consult your physician.

The rest of this book is dedicated to tips and tricks that you can use to change your habits, and possibly create new ones, in order to:

- fall asleep more easily
- stay asleep longer
- wake up feeling rested

I hope you are ready, because if you are suffering from a sleep disorder, you are about to receive the keys to the sleep castle. This is going to be a real game changer!

PART B

HOW TO SLEEP BET-TER

9. SEVEN SLEEP MYTHS DEBUNKED

"Laugh and the world laughs with you; snore, and you sleep alone!"

Anthony Burgess

9.1 Introduction

So far, we have covered the basics of sleep.

Let's recap what you have learned in 'Part A – Sleep Explained':

- Sleep is a natural recurring period of rest for the mind and body, in which we are not conscious, our voluntary muscles are relaxed, and our sensitivity to external stimuli is diminished.
- Although it is not entirely clear why we sleep, it is important to get enough sleep. Getting enough sleep is associated with benefits like improved health, mood and memory, whereas sleep deprivation negatively affects your health, mood and concentration.
- We sleep in cycles of approximately ninety minutes, which consist of two types of sleep: Non-Rapid-Eye-Movement (NREM) sleep and Rapid-Eye-Movement (REM) sleep.

- Your sleep/wake cycle is governed by an internal clock that makes you feel alert and sleepy. This circadian rhythm is not only influenced by natural factors, but also by external factors such as light, time and melatonin.
- Although a small percentage of the population are natural short sleepers, most of us will need to sleep seven to eight hours a night in order for the brain to flush out chemicals it does not need, and for the body to recharge.
- Dreams mostly occur in REM sleep. It is still a mystery why we dream. Yet we do know that being deprived of REM sleep causes all kinds of negative behavioral changes.
- A sleep disorder can have a detrimental impact on your life, causing a variety of health issues.

We have now arrived at the second part of this book: 'Part B – How To Sleep Better'. This part of the book is jam-packed with strategies, tips and tricks you can use to sleep more soundly.

But before we get into those, we need to first address a number of common sleep myths. Because in order to take effective action to improve the quality of your sleep, you need to first understand what does not work.

***

9.2 Sleep Myths

Have you ever tried counting sheep when you couldn't sleep? Or even masturbated?

With sleep being such an important part of life, it is surrounded by myths. There are all kinds of beliefs on how to fall asleep easily and have a good night rest. And while some of these may have a thin factual basis, many of them have not. Below we will tackle some of the most common misconceptions about sleep, and explain why they are false:

1. Counting sheep will help you fall asleep
2. Drinking alcohol before going to bed will help you sleep better
3. Old people need less sleep than young people
4. Masturbating helps you fall asleep more easily
5. When you are asleep, your brain rests
6. It is always better to get more sleep
7. On weekends you can make up for lost sleep

***

9.3 Sleep Myth #1: Counting Sheep Will Help You Fall Asleep

This myth has deep roots. It probably goes back thousands of years, to shepherds counting their sheep every day to check if any of them were missing. Even Jesus used counting sheep in one of his parables (Luke 15:4):

"Which of you men, if you had one hundred sheep, and lost one of them, wouldn't leave the ninety-nine in the wilderness, and go after the one that was lost, until he found it?"

It is likely that a shepherd would doze off occasionally while counting his sheep. But does that make it an effective technique for those that have difficulty falling asleep?

A study (goo.gl/WbfuhT) done by Oxford University's Department of Experimental Psychology suggests it is not. The subjects were divided in different groups, and they were asked to visualize different scenarios as they tried to fall asleep. One group was given no specific instructions.

The result? Those that counted sheep took up to twenty minutes longer to fall asleep than those who imagined other relaxing images scenarios such as a crackling fireplace!

The researchers concluded that visualizing these relaxing images takes up sufficient cognitive space to keep the person from engaging with distracting thoughts and concerns before falling asleep. Counting sheep on the other hand is probably too boring and repetitive to occupy enough cognitive space. This will make it easier for the person to re-engage with thoughts and worries, which in turn will make it more difficult to fall asleep.

***

9.4 Sleep Myth #2: Drinking Alcohol Before Going To Bed Will Help You Sleep Better

Ever been to a party, and after a couple of glasses of alcohol you felt like just rolling into your bed? And are you one of those that love a glass of wine before going to bed after a stressful day, to relax and unwind?

The good news is: yes, alcohol will help you fall asleep faster. But...you should still avoid drinking alcohol in the couple of hours before going to bed.

Here's why.

A 2013 study reviewing 27 scientific studies on the impact of drinking on sleep resulted in the findings that alcohol:

- indeed shortens the time it takes to fall asleep,
- also increases deep sleep,
- But...reduces REM sleep

And that is the catch.

If you remember, we sleep in NREM and REM cycles of approximately ninety minutes. And as the night progresses, the amount of REM sleep per cycle increases. So, while alcohol may help you fall asleep more easily, ultimately your sleep won't be as satisfying and restful as it could be. REM sleep is very important: it is the restorative part of our sleep cycle. Getting enough REM sleep also influences memory, whereas a lack of REM sleep can negatively impact your memory and concentration.

When commenting on this review, Chris Idzikowski, director of the Edinburgh Sleep Centre said: *"In sum, alcohol on the whole is not useful for improving a whole night's sleep. Sleep may be deeper to start with, but then becomes disrupted. Additionally, that deeper sleep will probably promote snoring and poorer breathing. So, one shouldn't expect better sleep with alcohol."*

There's nothing wrong with the occasional glass of alcohol. But if you habitually drink one or more glasses of alcohol in order to fall asleep more easily, you may want to rethink that habit.

As a rule of thumb, keep in mind that it is best not to drink any alcohol two to three hours before you go to bed.

***

9.5 Sleep Myth #3: Old People Need Less Sleep Than Young People

Another myth is that seniors need less sleep than younger adults.

Generally speaking, it is true that older people sleep less than their younger counterparts. But that is not because they need less sleep. As we age, our sleep patterns change. Older people find it harder to fall asleep, and awake more often during the night, and earlier. They wake up more often because they experience discomforts, or suffer from chronic pains. Also, they spend less time in deep, dreamless sleep.

So it is not that old people need less sleep. They just have more difficulty sleeping a full night because of their age, and the discomforts that come with it.

***

9.6 Sleep Myth #4: Masturbating Helps You Sleep Better

Until not too long ago, the topic of masturbation was taboo, and considered shameful. In conservative Christian circles, masturbating was even viewed as sinful. This is based on the story of Onan. He was put to death by God for spilling his semen on the ground, instead of fulfilling his duty to his deceased brother by entering into a levirate marriage with his brother's widow Tamar and give her offspring (Genesis 38:8-9).

Nowadays, scientists claim that masturbation comes with a number of health benefits, like preventing depression, lowering the risk of heart disease and reducing stress. But does it help you sleep better?

A 1985 study (goo.gl/CVus2S) on five men and five women showed that giving oneself a hand does not impact one's sleep:

"The analysis of several sleep parameters did not reveal any effect of masturbation on sleep. These results suggest that physiological changes that occur during masturbation, with

or without orgasm, have no major effect on sleep organization."

But what about falling asleep? Surely, with the release of endorphin and oxytocin hormones after the 'Big O' it will be easier to drift off into dreamland?

Contrary to what some popular blogs will want to make you believe, there is no scientific evidence for this. This does not mean it is not true, though. According to Nicole Prause, sex researcher and founder of Liberos, an independent research institute that studies orgasms, *"we don't actually know, because it's never been studied."*

There is however scientific research suggesting that consistent bedtime routines can improve the quality of sleep. And if pleasuring yourself before going to sleep is part of your bedtime routine, you may fall asleep shortly after orgasming because you believe masturbation helps you fall asleep more easily. But really it is the bedtime routine that does the trick.

***

9.7 Sleep Myth #5: When You Are Asleep, Your Brain Rests

When you go to sleep, you close the curtains and turn off the light. Similarly, you close your eyes and your brain turns off. Right?

Wrong.

When you fall asleep, you lose consciousness. But your brain remains active. The prime example is of course dreaming: feeling the wind in your hair flying through the sky on a purple unicorn, all while being chased by a crossover between Kermit the Frog and a Lily yelling at you with an Arnold Schwarzenegger accent "Get Over Here!", requires a lot of brain activity.

But there is more.

Sleeping helps in consolidating memories, which is crucial if you want to learn new information.

Learning new information happens in three phases:

1. Acquisition
2. Consolidation
3. Recall

The first and third only take place when you are awake. However, according to scientific research, consolidation of memories occurs when you are asleep. Our memories are formed through the strengthening of the neural connections during sleep.

One scientific study (goo.gl/pJTeCa) even showed that sleeping helps people in recovering skills that they had forgotten during the day. For a study conducted by the university of Chicago, two hundred college students were divided into four groups. Most of the students were women, with little previous experience playing video games.

They were asked to play the video game, without training. Next, they received training on how to actually play the video game, after which they played it again. Then, depending on which group they were in, they were asked to play the game another time, twelve and twenty-four hours later. At the twelve hour mark, they had not had any sleep yet (they played the video game in the morning, and then again in the evening), whereas they had a night of sleep at the and twenty-four hour mark.

As you would expect, the researchers found that the subjects had become more skillful at playing the game immediately after the training. However, much of that skill was lost after twelve waking hours. Then, when the students played the video game after a night of sleep, they showed a ten-percentage point improvement over their performance prior to the training.

When asked about these results, Howard Nusbaum, Professor of Psychology at the University of Chicago, and a researcher in the study said:

"The students probably tested more poorly in the afternoon because following training, some of their waking experiences interfered with training. Those distractions went away when they slept and the brain was able to do its work."

Why is this study interesting? Because it shows that lost skills are restored when you are asleep!

So while you are taking a break of your daily busy life, your brain actually helps you process that day, consolidates the information you have acquired, and prepares you for the next day.

How cool is that, huh?!

***

9.8 Sleep Myth #6: It Is Always Better To Get More Sleep

By now, you know that, unless you are a natural short sleeper, you should make sure that you get at least seven to eight hours of sleep every night. But is there a maximum? Is getting more sleep always better?

In Chapter 6 'How Much Sleep Do We Need', you learned that in a June 2015 Sleep Journal publication, the American Academy of Sleep Medicine (AASM) recommended at least seven or more hours of sleep per night for adults aged 18 to 60 years. But the AASM *"did not place an upper limit on recommended sleep duration, agreeing that sleeping more than nine hours per night on a regular basis may be appropriate for young adults, individuals recovering from sleep debt, and individuals with illnesses."* (goo.gl/yFR7lw)

So that doesn't tell us much. If sleeping eight hours is better than four, does that also mean that sleeping eleven hours is better than eight?

This doesn't seem to be the case. Franco Cappuccio, professor of Cardiovascular Medicine and Epidemiology at the University of Warwick, analyzed 16 studies on sleeping habits. Combined, more than a million people were involved as subjects in these studies. Cappuccio roughly divided these subjects in three groups:

- Subjects that slept less than six hours a night (short sleepers)
- Subjects that slept six to eight hours a night (medium sleepers)
- Subjects that slept more than eight hours a night (long sleepers)

When following up with these people, Cappuccio found that long sleepers are 30% more likely to die younger, compared to the medium sleepers.

It is still debated whether there is a direct causal link between sleeping too long and dying earlier. But after correcting the analysis for subjects using sleeping pills or being depressed, the result was still the same. Cappuccio theory is that long sleepers may have an underlying health problem, that isn't yet showing any other symptoms than sleeping longer.

However, a study by Shawn Youngstedt, professor at Arizona State University, suggests that the problem with sleeping longer is the prolonged physical inactivity.

He asked 14 young adults to stay in bed two hours more per night, for three weeks.
When asked about their experience, they complained about back pain and soreness, as well as increased bad moods.

So the jury is still out whether sleeping longer has detrimental effects on one's health. But the evidence so far suggests that you are better off if you kick into gear and get out of bed when you wake up in the morning.

***

9.9 Sleep Myth #7: On Weekends You Can Make Up For Lost Sleep

Most of us have a tendency to sleep in during the weekend, after a week of hard work and probably not enough sleep. But can you catch up with the Zzzs you missed out on?

According to Dr. W. Christopher Winter, of Charlottesville Neurology and Sleep Medicine, you can if you do so within a few days. But this is not a sustainable method for catching up with missed sleep over a long period of time.

When asked about this, dr. Chuck Smith, a care physician at the University of Arkansas for Medical Sciences, also confirmed that it is possible to catch up with some lost sleep in the weekend. However, he added that *"the amount of sleep lost and recovered may not be the same, though. Most of the first few hours of sleep can be recovered, but if the amount of sleep lost is more than a few hours, not all of it will be recovered."*

With that being said, if we are short on sleep our bodies have a way of bouncing back from sleep deficit. Our body is so well organized, that when it does catch up, it tries to recover as much of the REM sleep and deep sleep as possible, while skipping some of the other sleep stages. This means that we would not even need to recover all the missed hours.

Still, it is best to maintain a regular sleeping routine. One where you go to bed around the same time, and wake up the next morning around the same time, every day. Weekdays and weekends. This will give you the best sleep!

10. MAKE YOUR BEDROOM A SLEEP SANCTUARY

"I have the same bedroom I've always had. It's clean and tidy when I get home, and after two or three days it gets messy and my mother nags me."

Rafael Nadal

10.1 Introduction

Unless you are a monk who has trained his mind to stay equanimous regardless of the external circumstances, you are influenced by your surroundings. At least to a certain degree, most people will feel:

- moody, when it is cold and rainy
- uplifted and joyful, when the sun shines
- peaceful and relaxed, when they play with a puppy or kitten
- connected and appreciated, when they receive a hug from a loved one

Knowing this, it only makes sense that the way you have organized your bedroom is going to have an impact on how easily you fall asleep.

***

10.2 Your Bedroom Is Where You Go To Sleep

If somebody would put a gun to my head and told me that I was only allowed to give one tip to help people sleep better, or else…

I would give this advice: **keep anything that is not conducive to falling asleep out of your bedroom.**

This one piece of advice is so powerful! Actually, a lot of the tips and tricks that follow later on in this book are simply elaborating on this theme.

Why is it so important?

One word: Habit.

Although the brain only represents about 2-3 % of the weight of an adult, it consumes approximately 20% of the energy produced by the body. To use the body's energy most effectively, our brain is constantly looking for ways to reduce the amount of energy it consumes.

Enter habits.

A habit is a choice that we deliberately make at some point, and then stop thinking about, but continue doing, often every day. On autopilot.

Let's take driving a car, for example. And if you don't know how to drive a car, just think of riding a bicycle or even walking. No one knows how to drive when they are born into this world. So when you took your first driving lessons, all your senses were on. Both your hands were on the steering wheel. Your right feet on the gas pedal, your left foot alternating between resting, stepping on the clutch pedal, or hitting the brake. Your eyes were anxiously scanning the road ahead, or taking a sneak peek in the rear-view and wing mirrors. The radio was turned off, so you wouldn't miss any traffic sound that would possibly require you to slow down or speed up. All your energy was directed to driving that car!

Now fast-forward to a few years later. You're commuting to work, driving your car effortlessly. You're listening to Adele playing on the radio. At the same time, you're running the presentation you will give later today through your head. And, oh wait, you shouldn't forget to buy coffee beans on your way back home!

When you finally arrive at the office, you may even wonder: how did I get here, did I take road A or road B this time?

The reason why you arrived safely at work is because you've developed the habit of driving. Learning how to drive required your full attention. But once you had it figured out, you could almost do it on autopilot. And your brain freed up energy resources for other things it needs to process.

Studies show that 40-45% of everything we do on a daily basis is a habit. It happens automatically.

In his book 'The Power of Habit', which was on the New York Times best-seller list for two years, Charles Duhigg explains that every habit is a loop made up of 3 simple ingredients:

1. Cue
2. Routine
3. Reward

The cue is the trigger for an automatic behavior to start. The routine is the behavior itself. And the reward is what you get out of that behavior.

An example that Duhigg gives is the habit of eating a chocolate chip cookie every afternoon in the cafeteria. Without knowledge of how habits work, you might rely on your willpower to stop this behavior. However, studies suggest that willpower is a finite resource: it can be depleted. If you solely rely on willpower to make long-lasting changes, you will probably fail many times, and beat yourself up about it in the process.

A smarter move is to figure out the habit loop. First, you identify the routine. This is the behavior you want to change. In Duhigg's example: getting up in the afternoon, going to the cafeteria and eating the chocolate chip cookie.

And what is the reward? This may of course simply be the cookie. But it could also be the sugar spike that comes with eating a cookie, socializing with colleagues, or simply stretching your legs. The reward may not be immediately apparent, so you will probably have to experiment with different rewards, but you get the idea.

Finally, you need to figure out the cue for this routine: what triggers the urge to get up, buy a chocolate chip cookie and eat it? Maybe you get bored in the afternoon. Or you're hungry. Perhaps your blood sugar is low.

Once you've figured out what triggers the behavior, and what reward you get out of it, you can start working on shifting the behavior.

In case of the chocolate chip cookie, Duhigg figured out the reward was socializing with colleagues. So he set an alarm at 3:30 p.m. to go talk to a colleague for ten minutes. And though you don't change a habit overnight, eventually the new behavior becomes automatic, because you have left the cue and reward untouched.

So that is how habits work.

But what does all of this have to do with keeping any activity that is not related to sleeping out of your bedroom?

Well...everything!

If you make your bedroom an area designated for sleep (and sex) only, then to your brain this room becomes associated with the behavior of sleep (routine). Going to your bedroom to prepare for bed triggers that behavior (cue). And the reward is getting rest and waking up recharged (reward). Do this everyday, and you'll create a very powerful habit that is conducive to falling asleep more easily.

However, this does not work if you are more lenient with what types of behavior you allow in your bedroom. If you also:

- play video games
- exercise, or
- work on your laptop

in your bedroom, going to your bedroom can be the cue for any of these behaviors.

If you are serious about the quality of your sleep, and falling asleep more easily, your bedroom needs to be a sacred place. If it isn't an activity that is meant to be done in bed, it should not be allowed in your bedroom.

Sleep Hacks:

- **Review Your Bedroom Behaviors:** do you reserve your bedroom for sleep and sex only? Or are you playing video games, or working on your laptop?
- **Understand How Habits Work:** Be honest with yourself. You may think that what you do in the bedroom besides sleeping isn't really important. But that may simply be a matter of habit. Understand the power of signaling to your brain that you are going to sleep the moment you enter the bedroom.

- **Review Your Bedroom Habits**: Use the Cue/Routine/ Reward loop to analyze your bedroom habits.
- **Change Your Bedroom Habits**: If you spot a bedroom habit that isn't conducive to having a good night sleep, work on changing that habit. Keep in mind though that it takes time to change a habit, or even build a new one. They don't appear overnight. Be patient and compassionate with yourself if you fall back in an old habit. There is always a new day. Success is simply a matter of standing up one more time than you fall.

***

10.3 Keep Your Bedroom Calm And Clean

So it starts with using your bedroom for bedroom activities only. But there is much more you can do to make it crystal clear to your brain that this room has no other purpose than going to bed. Period.

Your bedroom should be a calm place associated with sleep and relaxation. It is well known that in order to be more productive, it helps to have a clean and organized desk. This creates space in the mind. The same holds true for falling asleep more easily. If you enter a room that is clean and organized, you will feel more relaxed. Perhaps having a calm and clean room won't matter so much after you have turned off the light and are lying in bed. But there is a phase before that, where you enter the bedroom and prepare for going to bed. It is easier to let go of the stress and the worries of the day if your bedroom is free of clutter. And the more relaxed you are, the easier you will fall asleep.

Don't have half of your clothes lying around your room, but store them in a closet. Ideally, your closet comes with doors that can be closed, so all those clothes and shoes are indeed completely out of sight.

Store any loose items under your bed. Most beds will have open space under it that you can use to store a bunch of non-essential stuff you don't regularly use. This could be anything: shoes, puzzles or games, or that extra blanket you only use in wintertime. Some beds come with built-in storage. If not, you could create your own, to make most efficient use of the space.

If you want to take it one step further, you can give your bedroom a more relaxing vibe by painting your walls in a tranquil color. This could be a cloudy shade of gray and blue, or soft coral. As long as it calms you, the exact shade doesn't matter that much.

It may also help to put up relaxing decorations on the wall. Whether it is a dream catcher above your bed, a photo of a loved one, or a relaxing piece of art: whatever works for you.

Besides creating a calm environment, it is also important to keep your bedroom clean. Not just to calm the mind, but also to improve the quality of your sleep. If you do not clean your room regularly, it will get dusty. Remember that you will inhale the air in your bedroom seven to eight hours a night, every night. So try to clean your bedroom at least once a week.

It is also crucial to ventilate your bedroom. Your bedroom should have at least one window that you can open and close. It would be best to sleep with the window opened slightly, so you can get a steady flow of fresh air throughout the night. But if that is not possible, for example because it is too cold or too noisy outside, at least ventilate your bedroom by having the window open during the day. It may also help to use a humidifier to improve air quality, or turn on a fan to improve circulation.

Sounds like a lot of work? If it does, think of the bigger picture here. The key message is that, in order to improve the quality of your sleep and fall asleep more easily, it helps to have a calm and clean bedroom. Once you have implemented these suggestions, with the exception of cleaning and ventilating your room, you don't need to think twice about them anymore.

There is no need to be a perfectionist here. Apply the 80/20 rule, also known as the Pareto Principle. This rule says that 80% of [some result] comes from 20% of [some cause].

Be practical. Keeping your room calm and clean doesn't mean you need to as far as organizing your books in a certain order.

Side note: this actually reminds of one of my former roommates, who organized all his books on his bookshelf according to size. The tallest books on the left side and the shortest books on the right side. One day, me and my other roommate decided to prank him and turned all the books in the reverse order: tallest on the right, shortest on the left. After my roommate got home, and we had dinner together, he didn't mention the books. At all. We waited. But he kept quiet in the following days too. So a couple of days later, when my roommate had left the house to attend a class, we went into his room again to check. And to our surprise, all the books had been put back into the original order...

Figure out which 20% of your actions can create 80% of the desired result: a calm and clean bedroom.

Sleep Hacks:

- **Do The Grandma Test:** walk into your room, imagining you are your grandma. Would she be impressed by how calm and clean your room is? Or would she feel the immediate urge to take out a mop and start cleaning it?
- **Ask Yourself: Does Entering Your Bedroom Make You Feel Relaxed?:** sometimes we cannot see the forest for trees anymore, because our bedroom is, well...that room where we spend one-third of every day, week in, week out. But if you are having trouble falling asleep, improving the calmness and cleanliness of your bedroom can have a great impact.
- **Keep Your Bedroom Organized**: store your clothes in a closet. Store other items under your bed.

- **Keep Your Bedroom Clean**: try to clean your bedroom at least once a week.
- **Turn Your Bedroom Into a Calm Environment**: paint your walls in a tranquil color. And put up relaxing decorations on the wall.
- **Ventilate Your Bedroom Daily**: ideally, sleep with an open window. If that is not possible, open the window during the day. Also consider installing a humidifier or a fan.
- **Don't Be a Perfectionist**: apply the 20/80 rule, where you identify the 20% of the changes that will have 80% of the desired result of having a clean bedroom that calms the mind when you enter it.

***

10.4 Keep Your Bedroom Cool

Have you ever been outside when it snowed, and then when you got back into your warm living room, sitting on the couch with a cup of hot chocolate, you started to feel sleepy? And perhaps you have also experienced the opposite: not being able to sleep while on a holiday, because of the high room temperature.

The temperature in your bedroom has a profound impact on your sleep quality. When tanning on the beach, 86°F / 30°C may be a great temperature. But not so in your bedroom!

Your body temperature rises and falls slightly during the day, reaching its lowest point around 5:00 a.m., after which it slowly starts to climb again. Your sleep cycle is tied to this pattern. Basically, when your body temperature starts to drop, you get drowsy. And a cool body optimizes release of melatonin, which is popularly called the sleep hormone. When it gets dark, the pineal gland in your brain will start to release melatonin. Melatonin prepares your body for sleep, and while you are asleep it allows your body to recuperate.

A tropical room temperature is not conducive to a good night sleep. Studies have found that the temperature of your bedroom affects your sleep quality more than outside noise. A moderate room temperature nudges your internal temperature down, resulting in a more restful and deep sleep.

Most sleep experts recommend a room temperature somewhere between 60°F and 68°F, or 16°C and 20°C. This helps the body's core temperature to drop, preparing you for sleep, according to a 2008 study published in the journal Brain (goo.gl/Xg7vZx). And keeping your bedroom well ventilated at night is even more helpful.

When adjusting your room temperature, also take your bed covers and pajamas into account: if your room temperature is just right, but you are wearing woolen socks in bed, lying under six thick blankets...well, you get the picture.

You may want to test which bedroom temperature is most comfortable for you. While the above room temperature advice is a good general guideline, ultimately what matters most is how you actually feel under the covers. You shouldn't feel hot or cold in bed, but just in that sweet spot in the middle. Therefore, consider keeping a sleep journal for a week, in which you score the quality of your sleep while trying out different room temperatures.

Side note: You don't want to overdo it with cooling down your room temperature. A couple of years ago, I moved apartments. My first apartment only had a fan to cool the air. And it wasn't even that powerful. As it was getting hotter and hotter, I found myself having trouble falling asleep. Luckily, my new apartment had air conditioning. On my first day, I turned the air conditioner on before I went to bed. I hadn't been in my apartment during the day, so the heat had built up and the room temperature was really high. So after a while, I decided to put the temperature down a few notches more. That did the trick, I fell asleep. But a few hours later I woke up again. As I slowly regained consciousness, I noticed I was shaking. And why was half my body covered in ice? Ok, there was no ice. But there might as well have been. I was freezing! I ended up drinking ginger tea for a week to alleviate my throat infection...

Sleep Hacks:

- **Check Your Bedroom Temperature:** what is the temperature in your bedroom when you go to sleep? And how do you feel when you are in bed: just right, or do you regularly feel too warm or too cold?
- **Test Which Bedroom Temperature is Most Comfortable For You**: for one week, keep a sleep journal. Score the quality of your sleep, while experimenting with different room temperatures.
- **Set Your Ideal Bedroom Temperature:** depending on your test results, adjust the room temperature to your liking. Be creative: consider installing an air conditioner, if you don't have one. Or keep the window open at night to ventilate the room. Alternatively, if your room is too cold, wear some pajamas and/or put an extra blanket on your bed.

***

10.5 Keep Your Bedroom Quiet

I remember being a teenager and going camping with my family in France. My parents slept in a trailer tent, while my siblings and me slept in small tents next to it. Soundproofing level? Zero. In the spot next to us, our neighbors enjoyed listening to the radio until deep in the night. At first, my dad asked them politely if they could turn it down. But even with the lower volume, it kept him out of his sleep, slowly driving him mad. A few days later we packed our stuff and moved to a different camping...

Studies have shown that external noise can have a great negative impact on sleep quality, possibly even resulting in long-term health issues. This is not the same for everyone. Some people just fall asleep within minutes after going to bed, and then sleep like a rock for the rest of the night.

> **Side note:** For example, one time my ex-girlfriend had decided she wanted to wake up at 7am. Being a notorious late sleeper, she had set seven (!) different alarms to go off over the course of two to three hours. One tip: if you are ever considering doing this, I highly recommend communicating this with your partner before going to bed...This night won't go down in history as one of my most restful nights! I woke up at 4:30 a.m., in slight panic, not understanding what was happening, and what that noise was. While my girlfriend was sound asleep, I had to roll over to her side of the bed and figure out how to turn off the alarm. And then when I had almost dozed off again, 20 minutes later the alarm went off again. And again...

But if you are reading this book, you are probably not one of those people that sleep like a baby all through the night. And if the problem was limited to only waking up...but once you are awake, it can take a long time before you fall asleep again. And if the sound is repetitive, you may not be able to fall asleep at all anymore!

To make sure it is quiet at night in your bedroom, start by picking the right location. Pick a quiet neighborhood. If external noise is an issue for you at night, do not rent an apartment that is located right above or close to a bar, a restaurant, or on a busy road.

Chances are however that you are stuck with what you have got. If you live in a house or apartment with multiple rooms, consider changing the location of the bedroom. Ideally, your bedroom is the furthest away from the external noise source. So if your house is located on a busy road, make sure your bedroom is in the back, and not on the side of road.

See if you can improve the isolation of the walls. This may not be an issue in houses that were built recently, but older houses tend to have bad sound isolation. The walls don't need to be soundproof, but isolating the walls can really make a difference.

The same goes for your windows. Although having a window open at night is good for ventilation, you need to close it if external noise is waking you up. If your window uses a single pane of glass, you may want to consider double or even triple glazing. This means that the window has two or even three glass windowpanes separated by a vacuum or gas filled space. The primary purpose is regulating the temperature. But a great side effect is that it also reduces external noise.

If applying these tips is impractical or simply impossible in your situation, or after applying them the external noise still keeps you out of your sleep, try balancing that noise, for example by turning on a fan. It does not only help with cooling your body temperature, but the whir of a fan can also be soothing, reducing the impact of distracting external noise. Or try a white noise machine. This is a device that typically produces a sound that sounds like wind blowing through the trees, or running water. Other soothing sounds that white noise devices designed to aid with falling asleep may produce are rain or wind. A fan or white noise machine can also be helpful if your room is completely silent. Although silence is what you aim for, when your bedroom is dead quiet, any sudden sound can be disruptive.

Last but not least, wear earplugs at night. Even the simplest $1 foam earplugs can make a great difference in keeping out distracting sounds.

You may even want to spend some money on buying noise-cancelling earplugs. This is still a developing niche market. In 2014, Hush raised $ 593,255 on Kickstarter to make wireless noise masking earplugs that connect to your phone via Wi-Fi. If you have ever tried premium noise-cancelling headphone (for years, Bose has been leading this market), you know how powerful the effect can be. Although the Amazon reviews of the Hush earplugs are mixed, if future noise-cancelling earplugs can deliver on their promise, they might be the solution to all external noise problems.

Sleep Hacks:

- **Live in a Quiet Neighborhood**: don't live next to a nightclub in the middle of the city if you are a light sleeper.
- **Make Sure Your Bedroom is as Far Away as Possible From the External Noise:** make sure your bedroom is in the back of the house, if the front side of your house is on a busy road.
- **Improve the Isolation of Your Bedroom Walls and Windows:** isolating your bedroom walls can make a great difference in keeping out distracting sounds. The same goes for double or triple glazing.
- **Turn on a Fan or a White Noise Machine:** the whir or a fan or white noise machine is not only soothing, but also reduces the impact of disruptive noises.
- **Wear Earplugs:** even the simplest foam earplugs can greatly improve the quality of your sleep. If you have some more money to spend, consider buying noise-masking earplugs.

***

10.6 Keep Your Bedroom Dark

When it gets dark, your pineal gland starts producing more melatonin, the sleep hormone. This sends the signal to your body that it is time to go to sleep. You start to feel drowsy and become less alert.

If you have difficulty falling asleep, making your bedroom as dark as possible can really help. Even though your eyelids are closed, some light is still able to pass through it. So the darker your bedroom, the better.

First, don't have any lights on at night, not even dimmed. And also don't have a digital alarm clock that gives off bright light. When you need to leave the bed at night, to go to the toilet for instance, do not turn on the lights. Use a flashlight or a infrared night-light. Turning on a bright light signals to your brain that it is time to wake up.

Next, use dark, heavy curtains. Or put up blackout shades. This is especially important if there is artificial lighting coming in from outside, like streetlight.

Finally, you may want to put on a sleep mask. Some people find wearing a sleep mask uncomfortable though, and actually have more difficulty falling asleep when they wear one. Do your own experiment, testing different sleep masks, and pick the one that is comfortable to you.

Sleep Hacks:

- **Make Your Bedroom as Dark as Possible**: turn off all lights, and use dark curtains or blackout shades.
- **Try Wearing a Sleep Mask**: though some people find wearing a sleep mask uncomfortable, it is great tool to block out any light.

11. TURN YOUR BED INTO A SLEEP HAVEN

"Self-pity in its early stage is as snug as a feather mattress.
Only when it hardens does it become uncomfortable."

Maya Angelou

11.1 Introduction

So far, we have discussed how you can improve the quality of your sleep by turning your bedroom into a calm and relaxing space.

However, we haven't touched on the most important part of your entire bedroom: your bed!

You can optimize every other part of your bedroom, but if you sleep on a bed of nails, chances are that you are not going to feel very rested and recharged when you wake up. If you can fall asleep at all…

***

11.2 Sleep On A Comfortable Mattress

It all starts with making sure your bed is equipped with a comfortable and supportive mattress. If you have slept on the same old mattress for many years, chances are that you will sleep much better simply by tossing that mattress away and buying a new one.

What is the best type of mattress? This is very subjective. A good mattress supports your body in a neutral position, one in which your body is aligned and your spine has a nice curvature. Although a hard mattress may be good for some people, this is definitely not the case for everyone! A mattress that is too firm may actually take you out of alignment. It all depends on your body, your sleeping habits, and the curvature of your spine. The best mattress for you is the one on which you feel no pressure.

Depending on the quality of your mattress, replace your mattress after seven to ten years. A good indication for replacing your mattress is when you wake up with back pain that you can get rid of merely by doing twenty to thirty minutes of yoga or stretching.

> *Tip:* To get started with yoga, check out my book 'Yoga For Beginners: 10 Super Easy Poses To Reduce Stress and Anxiety'. You can access it at here: amazon.com/ dp/B01N4ATAQY.

When you buy a new mattress, take your time to test it. When you visit a mattress store, don't hesitate to lie down and take some time to test a mattress. What are a few minutes compared to years of sleeping every night for seven to nine hours?! According to a 2016 survey conducted under 62,000 Consumer Reports subscribers, the more time people spent testing a mattress before buying, the higher their satisfaction. 77% of those that spent more than fifteen minutes were especially happy with their new mattress. So take your time: if you don't test the mattress, you might regret it later.

When buying a mattress online, and in many cases also when buying a mattress in a store, you are often allowed to return the mattress within a reasonable term and get your money back. So really keep track of your first nights on the mattress. Also make sure it actually fits in your bed.

It may take a few nights to get used to a new mattress. But if, after a few nights, you still feel this mattress is killing your back, don't hesitate to return it. Your health demands it.

Sleep Hacks:

- **Sleep On a Comfortable Mattress:** there is no such thing as a 'one size fits all mattress'. A good mattress for you is the one on which YOU feel no pressure. It supports your body in a neutral position.
- **Check In On How You Feel When You Wake Up:** how do you feel when you wake up in the morning? If you often experience back pain in the morning, this may be an indication that it is time to replace your mattress.
- **Replace Your Mattress After Seven To Ten Years:** a mattress does not have eternal life. If you have slept on your mattress for years, start looking for a new mat-

tress, especially if you wake up with physical discomforts.

- **Try Before You Buy:** when buying a new mattress, take the time to test it. Comfort is more important than price. Which mattress you buy is going to impact the quality of your sleep for years to come, so you do not want to make this decision lightly. If you do not test the mattress, you might regret it later.

***

11.3 Sleep Under A Warm Blanket And On A Comfortable Pillow

Having a good mattress is a great way to start. But to sleep like a baby, you also need warm blankets and a comfortable pillow to support your head.

How many blankets you use, and how thick they are, depends on the season. In general though, you are warm enough under your blanket(s), but do not overheat. If you feel stressed or anxious, you may even want to consider sleeping under a weighted blanket. Some people find these really soothing.

Pillows are like running shoes when you train for a marathon: perhaps the most important equipment for working out your Zzzs. Which pillow is best for you depends on your body, your sleeping position, and your personal preference. The key is to feel comfortable. Like with a mattress, you will want to test this.

A pillow that is too thick may push your head up to much. Whereas, if it is too thin, and you lie on your back, your head may tilt backwards. In both cases, you may wake up with a painful neck, which is something to avoid. And if you sleep on your belly, you may not even want to rest your head on a pillow at all, or use a very flat one.

Use just one pillow, don't pile up multiple pillows. This can mess up your body alignment, and can result in hurting your neck. A pillow should only support your head and neck, not your shoulders. What you want to aim for is finding a pillow that will keep your spine and neck in a straight line. This way, you avoid stress on your spine and neck, and you will fall asleep more easily.

If you suffer from chronic pains in your neck, you might be better off buying an orthopedic pillow with a scooped-out hollow. These pillows are designed to support your head and neck.

You can also use pillows to support other parts of your body. For example, if you sleep on your side, experiment with holding a pillow between your legs. Or if you sleep on your back, try placing a pillow under your knees. This can alleviate tension in your hips or lower back respectively.

Like with a mattress, a pillow that is past its due date can do more damage than good. So when should you replace your pillow? Every six months, says Robert Oexman, director of the Sleep to Live Institute, and definitely within two years, according to WebMD and the Sleep Council. It is always good to check in with how you feel. If you regularly start waking up with a painful neck, whereas this wasn't the case a year ago, it may be time to get yourself a new pillow.

Sleep Hacks:

- **Sleep Under a Warm Blanket:** the number and thickness of the blankets depends on the season. Make sure you are warm enough, but don't overheat.
- **Rest Your Head on a Comfortable Pillow**: which one is best depends on your body, sleeping position, and personal preference. Test before you buy.
- **Use Just One Pillow**: piling up pillows can cause tension on your neck and spine. Just use one pillow that comfortable supports your head and neck.
- **Use a Pillow to Support Other Parts of Your Body:** sleeping with a pillow between your legs, or under your knees can help alleviate tension in your hips or lower back.
- **Replace Your Pillow at Least Every Two Years**: a pillow that is past its due date can do more damage than good.

***

11.4 Use Your Bed For Sleep And Sex Only

Entering your bedroom in the evening should trigger a signal in your brain that it is time to go to sleep. To create this mind-set, you need to be strict about what activities you allow in your bed.

Let your bed be a sacred place: it is only meant for going to sleep, and having sex. Do not work on your laptop in bed, or watch TV. Don't even read a book in bed. These things stimulate your brain, and anything that stimulates you shortly before going to bed can potentially affect how quickly you fall asleep, and the quality of your sleep. If you consider reading before going to bed to be a sleep-inducing habit, at least experiment with reading your book outside your bed, for example sitting in a chair.

By doing so, you keep a clear distinction between which activities you allow to happen in your bed and which ones you don't. By building the habit of only using your bed for sleep and sex, you will train your brain to think this way, and it will eventually pick up on that.

Sleep Hacks:

- **Limit Your Bed Activities to Sleep and Sex Only**: by doing so, you send a strong signal to your brain that your bed is a sacred space for relaxation only.

***

11.5 Keep Pets Out

The soft purring sound of a cat lying on your chest, or cuddling up against you, can be a very relaxing experience. So is falling asleep with Fido besides you a good idea?

It depends.

Pets can be the greatest bed hogs. Although having your cat or dog close by may help you unwind or feel safe, having them in the same room can be detrimental to the quality of your sleep.

In a study by the Mayo Clinic conducted under 150 of their patients, 49% reported having pets. 56% of these pet owners allowed their pets to sleep in the bedroom, with 20% of those describing their pets as disruptive.

However, 41% of the pet owners perceived sleeping with their furry friends as unobtrusive or even beneficial to sleep.

It very much depends on your pet's nightly behavior. But if are having trouble falling - and staying - asleep, you may want to rethink sleeping with your pet in the bedroom.

Pets can bring unwanted allergy triggers into your bedroom, such as pollen, fleas, fur or dander, resulting in sneezing and itchy, watery eyes.

And have you ever noticed that your cat just likes to chill on the couch all day? That is because cats are nocturnal animals.

To see what cats can be up to at night, check out the fascinating BBC documentary 'The Secret Life of the Cat'. For this documentary, the makers tracked the nightly whereabouts of fifty cats in a small village, by attaching GPS and micro cameras to them. Spoiler alert: they are not sleeping!

So chances are that if you fall asleep with your kitty in the room, you will wake up a few hours later because she decided to go on an adventure. Or even if she stays put, you might find your cat wagging its tail up and down. In your face.

Also, some people like to sleep with the door closed. However, cats need to pee at night. Trust me, you don't want to wake up finding out your cat peed on your mattress.

If you have a dog, he might keep you awake with his snoring and snorting. Or he might jump on top of you at 5am because he is all excited about going out for a walk. There are plenty of funny YouTube videos showcasing how Fido is told to go back to sleep, and keeps coming back five minutes later, time and time again, hoping that THIS time you will magically have a change of heart, jump out of bed and go out for a walk.

If you cannot get yourself to remove your dog from your bedroom, for example because you feel safe knowing that your pup is sleeping right next to you, let him sleep in a crate next to your bed, instead of in your bed.

Sleep Hacks:

- **Ask Yourself if Your Pet Cuts Your Sleep Short:** sure, you love falling asleep with your furry friend besides you. But does your dog or cat regularly wake you up in the middle of the night?
- **If So, Keep Your Pet Out of The Bedroom**: this may take some time to get used to, both for you and your pet. Don't give in to the temptation to bring your pet back in the bedroom. Improving the quality of your sleep is the most important, and you will both get used to the new situation eventually. Plus, a little time apart has never hurt a relationship. You and your pet will be super excited to see each other the next morning!
- **Consult an Animal Trainer or Vet**: if your pet is having a lot of trouble adjusting to the new situation, considering asking your animal trainer or vet to help your pet transition to sleeping happily elsewhere in the house.

***

11.6 Check For Allergies

Do you regularly sneeze lying in bed, have a runny nose, feel itchy, and wake up feeling exhausted in the morning? And it is not just a cold, or pollen season? Then chances are that there are allergens in your bedroom triggering these symptoms.

If you are sleeping with your pet, try keeping him or her out of the bedroom for a week and see if that makes a difference.

If the symptoms remain, have a look around your bedroom: when is the last time you cleaned it, and washed your bed linens? Clean your bedroom and bed linens at least once a week.

Otherwise, you might suffer from a dust mite allergy. Before taking drastic measures, take a skin prick test. This is a test where your physician will prick a tiny bit of different allergens, like dust mite or pollen, on the surface of your skin. The skin will start to swell and turn red at the test spot if you are allergic to that particular substance.

If a dust mite allergy is indeed established, it is time to vigorously clean your room, and keep it clean. Anything that can contain dust mites needs to be kept clean, or even replaced.

An old mattress for example can contain up to two and a half times the amount of dust mites than a brand new one. And the same goes for pillows. So you might want to start by replacing them.

Make sure you also encase your bedding with dust mite covers. It is an illusion to think that your bedroom can be completely dust mite free. But dust mites feed off the flakes of your skin, and if you cut off their food supply, you are going to greatly diminish their number. You can even consider buying a hypoallergenic mattress and pillows, because this material is naturally dust mite resistant.

Wash your bed linens in hot water at least once every week.

Also consider removing all your carpeting, and replacing it with a hard floor. Vacuum your floor regularly, and use a HEPA (which stands for 'high efficiency particulate air') vacuum cleaner.

The key thing to remember is that keeping your bedroom clean lowers the number of dust mites.

Sleep Hacks:

- **If You Have Allergy Symptoms, Keep Your Pet Out and Clean Your Bedroom**: pets carry around allergy triggers like fleas or pollen. Also, accumulated dust can affect your respiratory system.
- **If the Symptoms Remain, Take an Allergy Test**: within minutes after taking it, a skin prick test will show you if you have any type of allergy.
- **Vigorously Clean Up Your Room if You Have a Dust Mite Allergy**: dust mites feed of skin flakes. A good place to start is replacing your bedding, and encase it with dust mite covers. Also replace your carpet for a hard floor. After that, it is a matter of keeping your room clean. Clean your bedding at least once a week with hot water, and your floor with a HEPA vacuum cleaner.

***

11.7 Make Your Bed Every Morning

Part of keeping your bedroom a sacred space that is designated for relaxation only, is making your bed every morning. It only takes a couple of seconds to make your bed, but you will sleep better as a result. According to a sleep survey conducted by the National Sleep Foundation, at least.

When asked whether they made their beds, 71% of the respondents reported that they made their bed (almost) every day. And those respondents were more likely to then say they had a good night's sleep (almost) every day compared to those that did not make their bed.

By making your bed in the morning, you send a signal to your brain that you are going to start your day. You are not sliding back in. And when you enter your bedroom in the evening and see a made up bed, it calms the mind. Your body knows it is time to shut your eyes and doze off when lying down.

In his 2014 commencement speech at The University of Texas at Austin, Naval Admiral William H. McRaven recalled having to make his bed to perfection every day during his six months of SEAL training. At the time he considered it to be a little ridiculous, since they were training to become fighting machines. But over time the wisdom of the simple act of making one's bed has proved its value to him many times over. He said:

"If you make your bed every morning, you will have accomplished your first task of the day. It will give you a small sense of pride, and it will encourage you to do another task, and

another, and another. And by the end of the day, that one task completed will have turned into many tasks completed.

Making your bed will also reinforce the fact that the little things in life matter. If you can't do the little things right, you'll never be able to do the big things right.

And if by chance you have a miserable day, you will come home to a bed that is made. That you made. And a made bed gives you encouragement that tomorrow will be better. So if you want to change the world, start by making your bed."

Sleep Hacks:

- **Make Your Bed Every Morning**: this will improve the quality of your sleep. It will also be your first completed task, kick starting a productive day. And if your day didn't go as planned, at least you can come home to nicely made bed, and start anew tomorrow.

***

11.8 Tips For Sleeping With A Partner

If you are like many other people, you enjoy cuddling with your partner in bed in order to unwind after a stressful day, culminating in dozing off to dreamland or taking that intimacy one
step further into making love.

But what if your partner is a real bed hog, turning around in his sleep all the time, stealing all the blankets, perhaps even kicking his or her legs?

To tackle this, instead of using a single set of bed covers, try two separate sets of sheets and duvets. This allows you to still do all the fun stuff. But when you go to sleep, it is less likely that your partner will wake you up. This is also great if one partner wants to sleep under just a thin bed sheet, whereas the other would like to wrap him- or herself up under a couple of blankets. If you are worried about how this might look to outsiders, you can simply cover your bed with a single comforter when making the bed in the morning.

This should help if your partner moves a lot at night. But what if your partner snores so loud that you are afraid the windows are going to break?

This is a real problem, one that many couples have to deal with. If the snoring is not too loud, and happens only occasionally, sleeping with earplugs could make all the difference. Or try to elevate the head of your bed, for example by putting some books under the legs at the head of your bed. This elevates the torso and could reduce snoring. Also, if your partner is not the type of person that moves a lot in his sleep, see if you can get him to sleep on his side. Snoring often happens when a person is sleeping on his back.

If this does not help, I recommend contacting a physician. People who snore heavily often have sleep apnea, which is a common disorder in which one's breathing is interrupted repeatedly throughout the sleep cycle. One of the symptoms is loud snoring. This is not only annoying for a partner, but also potentially dangerous for the person with the apnea, depending on how obstructed the airway is. Nowadays, you can spend a night sleeping in the hospital, under surveillance. Subsequently, the physician will discuss the results and give a recommendation on how to deal with this disorder. I will discuss this in more detail in Chapter 15 'Other Strategies To Improve Sleep Quality'.

Ultimately, if all else fails, consider sleeping in a different room. While this may not be the most romantic option, consider the alternative: if you are woken up every night because of your partner's snoring, you are going to feel grumpy and project this on your partner, which could potentially result in ending the relationship.

Sleep Hacks:

- **If Your Partner is a Bed Hog, Try Separate Sheets and Duvets**: you can still cuddle before falling asleep, but when you go to sleep it is less likely that your partner's movements will wake you up.
- **If Your Partner Snores, Try Earplugs First, and Otherwise Visit a Physician**: snoring can be an indication of sleep apnea, so it is a good idea to have a physician take a look at it and recommend what steps to take. If nothing helps, sleeping in another room might be your last option.

***

11.9 The Best Sleep Position

What is the best way to sleep? This is highly subjective. Often, when we can't fall asleep, we start twisting and turning, in the hope that this new position will do the trick.

Whatever sleep position you are in, set the intention to keep both your head and neck straight. This will improve the quality of your sleep. Don't sleep on your stomach though. This twists your neck, and can result in waking up with aches and pains. And if you cannot help yourself because lying on your stomach is just what puts you to sleep, at least experiment with placing your pillow under your hips instead of under your head.

Also consider changing into your birthday suit. Studies show that there are many benefits to sleeping naked. For starters, it helps regulate your body temperature, according to sleep specialists at the Cleveland Sleep Clinic. A lower skin temperature increases the quality of your sleep, and lowers the number of times you wake up, according to researchers at the University of Amsterdam. Moreover, sleeping naked has been shown to reduce stress and speeding up the body's metabolism, causing you to lose weight faster.

Sleep Hacks:

- **Whatever Sleep Position You Are in, Set the Intention to Keep Your Head and Neck Straight**: this will improve the quality of your sleep.
- **Try Sleeping Naked**: numerous studies have shown the health benefits of sleeping naked, such as sleeping more deeply and reducing stress.

12. GET YOUR LIGHT FIX DURING THE DAY, DIM THE LIGHTS AT NIGHT

"I remember being on a black-and-white set all day and then going out into daylight and being amazed by the color."

Jeff Bridges

12.1 Introduction

Artificial light exposure between dusk and the time you go to sleep suppresses the release melatonin, the sleep hormone. If you have trouble falling asleep, you will want to reduce your exposure to light in the hours leading up to bedtime. At the same time, you want to make sure expose yourself to enough natural light during the day.

***

12.2 Lower Your Exposure To Light In The Evening

To smoothen the transition between day and night time, start dimming the lights in the evening. Or if you don't have a dimmer, change a few light bulbs to a lower wattage. If you are reading this book on an e-reader (like Kindle), reduce the brightness.

Eliminate all other sources of light in your bedroom. So no digital alarm clocks, no digital photo frame, no lava lamps. Be vigorous here! If you cannot remove an item, for example because your air conditioner has a led light indicating the temperature, cover it. Try a piece of paper with tape, or a cloth cover. Use whatever you have available.

You can also experiment with using only natural light in the late evening, like lighting candles, or light a fire in a fireplace. Just make sure you turn off the candles or put out the fire before going to bed!

Sleep Hacks:

- **Dim the Lights**: dim the lights in the evening, or change a few light bulbs to a lower wattage.
- **Eliminate All Sources of Light in Your Bedroom**: remove or cover any sources of artificial light in your bedroom.
- **Experiment With Natural Light**: light candles or a fire.

***

12.3 Increase Your Exposure To Natural Light During The Day

The flipside of lowering your exposure to light in the evening is increasing your bright light exposure during the day.

This starts when you wake up and open the curtains. If you have no artificial light coming in at night through your windows, you may even want to keep your curtains open. This way, natural light can come in when the sun starts rising.

By letting the daylight in, you start suppressing the release of melatonin, in order to feel more alert and start your day. Nothing triggers waking up more than bright light. Well, a bucket of cold water in your face helps too. But seeing the sun is a much more pleasant way to wake up, wouldn't you agree?

Your body's internal biological clock, or circadian rhythm, regulates when you feel awake and sleepy. By reducing light exposure at night and increasing your light exposure during the day you keep your circadian rhythm in check. This will improve the quality of your sleep, and make you feel more energized during the day.

The more exposure to natural (sun)light you can get during the day, the better. Commuting to work? Try cycling or walking. Coffee or lunch break? Take a walk around the office. These little bits all add up in maintaining a healthy sleep-wake cycle.

Sleep Hacks:

- **Expose Yourself to Daylight as Soon as You Wake Up:** bright daylight sends a strong message to your brain that it's time to wake up.

- **Have a Break? Go Outside:** whenever you have time during the day, take that opportunity to go outside. These little bits of daylight exposure add up over the day and keep your circadian rhythm healthy.

13. STAY AWAY FROM ELECTRONIC DEVICES IN THE EVENING

"I don't have my iPhone or my iPad or anything in the bedroom. I do not, an hour before, or two hours before, get into some heavy kind of debates about business and stuff like that, or accept phone calls where those kind of things can happen. Because I've seen that then you go to bed and your mind keeps going and going and going and doesn't allow you to go to sleep. It's important to not do that."

Arnold Schwarzenegger, The Tim Ferriss Show #216

13.1 Introduction

In last decades, we have seen an explosion of electronic devices finding their way into our lives. The serial entrepreneur and CEO of Vayner Media Gary Vaynerchuk even argues that the smartphone is the new TV, and that right now we are seeing a transition from TV to phone similar to that from the radio to TV in the twentieth century. The difference is that our phone is always available, wherever we are. We have quickly developed into a society where it is normal, and in some businesses even expected, to be available 24/7.

Mobile phones have improved our lives in so many ways.

For example, in 2000, I attended a three-day music festival with 60,000 people. On the last day I lost my friends. And since none of us had a mobile phone at the time, trying to find each other was like searching for a needle in a haystack. I ended up roaming the fields on my own, and didn't see them again until later in the week, back home. Nowadays, a few WhatsApp message would have brought us back together.

Also, when you are traveling, you will never get lost again as long as you have Google Maps and GPS activated on your phone.

However, the constant stream of notifications and sensory stimulation that come with using a smartphone, or any other electronic device for that matter, is not conducive to good sleep. Therefore, you need to be mindful of how you use them.

***

13.2 Turn Off Electronics

It is a good idea to turn off all your electronic devices at least thirty minutes, or even better: one hour, before heading to bed.

This way, you put a halt on the continuous stimulation of your mind that happens all day long. Our mind isn't something that you can simply turn on and off. It is not a light switch.

If you are working on some spreadsheet on your laptop, or scrolling through your Facebook newsfeed on your smartphone, right before going to bed or even when you are in bed, how likely do you think it is that you'll be in a tranquil state and off to dreamland in minutes after turning those devices off? And the same goes for watching an episode of Game of Thrones on TV! When you turn off your electrical devices an hour before going to sleep, you give your mind the opportunity to unwind before going to sleep. And your sleep quality will be better as a result.

In 2011, the National Sleep Foundation (NSF) published the results of their Sleep in America® poll. They found that many Americans are sleep deprived, and that 95% of the people surveyed uses some type of electronics within the hour before going to bed. And mind you, this was only shortly after the introduction of the very first iPad, in 2010. It is safe to assume that use of (mobile) electronic devices is even more popular nowadays.

Commenting on the poll results, Charles Czeisler, PhD, MD, Harvard Medical School and Brigham and Women's Hospital, said:

"Artificial light exposure between dusk and the time we go to bed at night suppresses release of the sleep-promoting hormone melatonin, enhances alertness and shifts circadian rhythms to a later hour—making it more difficult to fall asleep. This study reveals that light-emitting screens are in heavy use within the pivotal hour before sleep. Invasion of

such alerting technologies into the bedroom may contribute to the high proportion of respondents who reported that they routinely get less sleep than they need."

We live in such a visual world, where we are online all the time, that it may sound hard and even crazy to turn of your electronic devices an hour before bedtime. But if you do, you will thank yourself for it in the morning, when you wake up rested, and refreshed. And it does not stop there. If you had a good, undisturbed sleep, you will find that you are able to concentrate better, and that the urge to take an afternoon nap is lower.

So give it a try! It may take a few evenings for your body and mind to adjust, but soon you will see your sleep quality improve.

Sleep Hacks:

- **Establish an Electronic Curfew**: one hour before you go to sleep, turn off your television, phone, laptop, and any other electrical devices.

***

13.3 Reduce Exposure To Blue Light

There is another reason why you will want to turn of your electronic devices completely, an hour before going to bed.

The blue light emanating from the screens of a tablet, smart-phone, or any other screen, messes up the body's natural circadian rhythm when exposed to it at night. This blue light suppresses the production of melatonin, a hormone that helps you sleep better. From an evolutionary perspective, bright light is a trigger for our brain that it is daytime. A time to be alert and awake. Moreover, the blue light stimulates the brain, and as we just discussed, you will want to allow for time for your brain to unwind.

It would be best to close your computer a couple of hours before you go to bed, and then keep it in another room, together with your phone and other electronics.

But if that is too hardcore for you, at least reduce the effect of the blue light of the screens. Luckily, these days there are apps that warm up your screen at night with a soft reddish color, which is much more gentle on the eyes. Once you set your time zone, these apps will automatically adapt the color of your screen as the night falls. F.lux is one of the most well known apps that allows you to do this. And Apple's IOS devices come with a similar feature called Night Shift.

So if you have to look at your tablet right before going to bed, at least make sure you install one of these apps!

Sleep Hacks:

- **Limit Your Exposure To Blue Light:** turn off your electronic devices a couple of hours before you go to bed, and keep them another room.
- **If This Is Too Hardcore, At Least Install F.lux or a Similar Color Filter App to Reduce Your Exposure To Blue Light:** the filtered colors are easier on the eyes, making it easier to fall asleep later. keep your electronics in another room, use a color filter app, or reduce the brightness. You can also reduce the brightness on your device.

***

13.4 Don't Talk On Your Mobile Phone Before Bed

Research suggest that calling on a mobile phone may negatively influence the production of melatonin, a hormone that induces sleep. This is due to the low-level radiation coming from the phone. Although this is not a scientific fact carved in stone, if you are struggling with falling asleep and need to make a call before going to bed, you may want to put it on speaker phone, or take the call on a landline.

Set the intention to not have any phone calls at all an hour before going to sleep. This will help ease the transition from a busy day to a tranquil state in which you can nod off easily.

Sleep Hacks:

- **Don't Hop on Phone Calls an Hour Before Going to Sleep:** doing calls just before bedtime may negatively influence the production of melatonin, and also doesn't help in calming your mind.

***

13.5 Set Your Phone To Silent Mode

In eastern spirituality, there is an expression that our mind is like a drunk monkey stung by a scorpion. Do you picture it?

You wouldn't want to try to fall asleep with that monkey in your room...

So it is important that you give your mind and body time so slow down in preparation for visiting la-la land.

If for whatever reason you cannot get yourself to turn off your electronic devices, at least set your phone to silent mode, and turn off notifications. This way you are only focused on one thing at a time. Even if that is watching House of Cards.

Sleep Hacks:

- **Set Your Phone Mute To Silent Mode:** if you can't get yourself to turn off your electronic devices, at least turn your phone on mute, to prevent getting distracted or woken up.

14. CHANGE YOUR DIET

"We want to do a lot of stuff; we're not in great shape. We didn't get a good night's sleep. We're a little depressed. Coffee solves all these problems in one delightful little cup."

Jerry Seinfeld

14.1 Introduction

What we eat and drink can affect our energy levels during the day, and the quality of our sleep at night.

Reviewing your dietary habits and experimenting with making some changes can really boost the quality of your sleep.

***

14.2 Avoid Eating Heavy Meals in the Evening

Eating a heavy meal just before going to bed is almost a recipe for sleeping badly. Eating a pizza at 11 p.m. overloads your digestive system, while your body is not meant to digest food during sleep. Digesting food takes a lot of energy, and you do not want to be doing this at a time where your body is meant to recharge.

Don't go to bed hungry, but stick to not eating anything two hours before going to bed. If you must eat something in the evening, opt for lighter snacks. There are studies suggesting that eating a meal with a lot of carbohydrates a couple of hours before going to sleep may help you nod off more easily. So eating a cracker with some cheese isn't all that bad. Just don't eat ten of them.

Have your biggest meal early in the day, breakfast or lunch. And make sure to include foods that are rich in magnesium and tryptophan, such as:

- Turkey
- Almonds
- Bananas
- Pumpkin seeds
- Green leafy vegetables, such as spinach
- Cherries
- Seafood, such as tuna and shrimp

These are just a few suggestions. It is best to do your own research and experiment with the types of food that work best for you.

In general though, consuming mostly unprocessed foods and cutting down on processed foods will improve the quality of your sleep. However, avoid spicy foods. Not only can they raise your body's temperature, but they can also keep you awake with heartburn.

You may even want to try intermittent fasting, where you only eat in an eight-hour window every day, for example between

11 a.m. and 7 p.m. This way you limit the time frame in which the body metabolizes the food.

And if you cannot get all the nutrients your body needs through the food you eat, take vitamins (B6 and B12), magnesium, calcium, and iron supplements.

Sleep Hacks:

- **Avoid Eating Heavy Meals in the Evening**: your body is meant to recharge during sleep, not digest food.
- **Don't Eat Anything Two Hours Before Going to Sleep**: don't go to bed hungry. But by making sure you consume enough calories during the day, you won't need to eat anything in the hours preceding sleep, and it will make falling asleep easier.
- **Include Foods in Your Diet That Are Rich in Magnesium and Tryptophan**: these can be found in foods like turkey, green leafy vegetables and bananas. Eating these foods during the day will help induce sleep at night.

***

14.3 Drink Enough Water

Keeping hydrated during the day is important, drink at least two liters of water. Drinking a big glass of water first thing in the morning boosts your metabolism, especially if you mix in some limejuice. Drinking enough water during the day also aids with weight loss, energizes your brain and let's you sleep more soundly.

However, like with food, avoid drinking any liquids two hours before going to bed. A sip of tea is okay, but if you jug down a liter of water just before going to bed, you will almost certainly wake up at night to pee. And before you know it, it takes an hour before you fall asleep again, making you feel low on energy the next day. So take it easy on liquids in the evening, and visit the bathroom before heading to bed.

If you want to drink something, sip on something warm. Try chamomile tea, or herbs like lemon balm, sage or valerian. These can help reduce anxiety and bring about sleep.

Sleep Hacks:

- **Drink Two Liters of Water Every Day:** drinking enough water energizes your entire system, and lets you sleep deeper.
- **Don't Drink Any Liquids Two Hours Before Going to Sleep:** drinking liquids before bedtime can result in waking up to urinate. If your mouth runs dry late at night, sip on a cup of herbal tea. And go to the bathroom before heading to bed.

***

14.4 Don't Consume Caffeine After 2 p.m.

For many people, their day does not really start until they have their first cup of Joe. The caffeine in a single cup of coffee can boost your energy, enhance focus, and overall performance. And it just tastes so darn good...

However, drinking too much coffee can significantly worsen the quality of your sleep. Caffeine is a stimulant that can prevent you from sleeping soundly, or even keeping you up in bed. It can stay in your system for as long as six to eight hours!

Therefore, do not consume any caffeinated drinks and foods after 2 p.m. And this is not limited to just coffee. Caffeine can also be found in cola, tea, chocolate, some pain relievers and weight loss pills.

If you do crave a cup of coffee later in the day, go for a decaf. Or switch to water or herbal tea.

Cutting coffee from your diet all together might be even better. If you cannot do without your daily shot of caffeine, try drinking tea instead. Tea also contains caffeine, but in a much smaller dose.

Sleep Hacks:

- **Don't Consume Caffeine After 2 p.m.**: caffeine is a stimulant that can stay in your system for six to eight hours. It is fine to drink coffee in the morning. But don't consume any caffeine later in the day, so your Zzzs are not affected.

***

14.5 Don't Drink Alcohol In The Evening

If drinking coffee is borrowing time from later in the day, drinking alcohol is a way of borrowing energy from tomorrow. And it is a loan on which you will have to pay interest.

Occasionally, this may be a price you are willing to pay. But if you care about sleeping well, make it a habit of not drinking alcohol in the evening. Although that glass of wine can shorten the time it takes to fall asleep, it can interfere with your sleep. It not only increases the likelihood of snoring, but also reduces REM sleep, resulting in feeling less energized than you could be when you wake up.

Sleep Hacks:

- **Don't Drink Alcohol Before Going to Sleep**: you may fall asleep more easily, but it comes at a cost: alcohol interferes with your sleep by reducing REM sleep, leaving you feeling less rested and recharged in the morning.

***

14.6 Quit Smoking

Like caffeine and alcohol, nicotine is a stimulant that can disrupt your sleep pattern.

Besides all the health risks associated with smoking, it can also make it more difficult to fall asleep. Moreover, smoking exacerbates sleep apnea. And smokers can experience withdrawal symptoms during the night, as their body craves nicotine. As a result, according to a 2008 study, smokers are four times as likely as nonsmokers to feel unrested after a night's sleep.

If you are a smoker, you may respond: *"Well, if I quit smoking I won't get any sleep!"* But you need not worry about that. The withdrawal symptoms you may experience when trying to quit smoking pass after about three days, after which your sleep pattern will normalize.

If you want to have a more restful sleep, kick your smoking habit, or at least reduce the number of cigarettes you smoke per day.

Sleep Hacks:

- **Quit Smoking**: nicotine is a stimulant that can keep you awake and leave you feeling unrested in the morning.

15. OTHER STRATEGIES TO IMPROVE SLEEP QUALITY

"There is a time for many words, and there is also a time for sleep."

Homer

15.1 Introduction

We have covered the most important strategies and hacks to sleep better.

You now know how to:

- make your bedroom into a sleep sanctuary
- turn your bed into a sleep haven
- increase your exposure to light during the day, and limit it in the evening
- limit your access to electronic devices at night, and
- make fundamental changes to your diet

Just by implementing the sleep hacks we have discussed so far in 'Part B - How To Sleep Better', you will sleep so much more soundly.

But we are going out with a BANG: in this chapter, you will learn a variety of other strategies are really the icing on the cake when it comes to sleeping well!

***

15.2 Exercise Regularly

One of the best ways to improve your sleep quality is regular exercise. A few hours after finishing your workout, your parasympathetic nervous system will take control and slow everything down, making you feel more relaxed. Your body will start to cool down, signaling the pineal gland to release melatonin, which will make you feel drowsy and wanting to go to sleep.

The beneficial effects of exercise on sleep quality have been shown by numerous studies. For example, in 2010, Northwestern Medicine performed a study on the effect of exercise on the sleep quality of a group of sedentary adults aged 55 and older, many of whom suffered insomnia. After sixteen weeks of doing aerobic exercises a few times per week, participants reported that their sleep quality had improved from poor to good. And as a bonus, they also reported fewer depressive symptoms, more vitality and less daytime sleepiness.

Exercise can be a real game changer for those that struggle with getting a good night sleep. What type of exercise doesn't really matter. Although your best option is vigorous exercise that pumps up your heart rate, any form of exercise is better than no exercise at all. High interval training, swimming, running, yoga, or even walking: they all help in getting better sleep. And even just five minutes of daily exercise can already help improve your sleep quality.

The key takeaway is that you need to exercise regularly, preferably every single day. If you have a strong gym routine, it is good to take daily breaks every now and then and give your body a rest. But going for a walk, or riding a bike, can be done on any day. The same is true when you are not in the best physical shape. Start with what you can do, and over time you will be able to improve your performance.

Don't exercise too close to bedtime though. In the hours after exercising, even though your body is tired, you will likely feel very energetic, making it impossible to fall asleep. The stimulatory effect of exercise increases alertness and the secretion of the hormone epinephrine (also known as adrenaline).

The rule of thumb is to finish your workout about four hours before hitting the sack.

If you want to do any exercise before going to bed, practice gentle exercises that focus on creating a mind-body connection, like Qi Gong, Tai Chi, or gentle yoga. These are slow practices that help calm the mind and relax the body, helping you to sleep longer and more soundly.

Sleep Hacks:

- **Exercise Daily**: you don't need to perform at the level of an Olympic athlete in order to improve the quality of your sleep. What is most important is having a routine where you exercise regularly, ideally every day. Acknowledge the level where you are at now, and start building your fitness from there.
- **Don't Do Vigorous Exercise Within Four Hours of Going to Bed:** although you may be the exception to the rule, most people will feel very energetic and awake in the first hours after finishing their workout. Therefore, it is best to not do any strong exercise shortly before going to bed.
- **Practice Gentle Exercises That Bring About Relaxation Instead**: exercises like Qi Gong, Tai Chi or gentle yoga connect mind and body and will help you to feel more relaxed. Check out my book 'Yoga For Beginners: 10 Super Easy Poses To Reduce Stress and Anxiety' to learn ten easy beginner techniques that will help release stress and anxiety, making you feel more relaxed and fall asleep more easily. Link: amazon.com/dp/B01N4ATAQY

***

15.3 Stick To A Sleep Schedule

Go to bed and wake up at roughly the same time every day. Also on weekends. Sleeping in on a Saturday may be tempting, but it will disrupt your biological clock. Your body cannot differentiate between work- and weekend days. Going to bed and waking up at different times can have the same effect on your internal clock as travelling across a few time zones.

And besides feeling jetlagged, if you go to bed at different times, drink alcohol and eat snacks on one night, then play Tetris on your phone just before bedtime another night, you are also missing out on a powerful tool to sleep better. Remember what we discussed earlier in Chapter 10, about the ingredients of habit? If you don't stick to a regular sleep schedule, the cue that could trigger the routine has no effect, because there is no automatic behavior. This does not mean of course that you can never deviate from your routine. But to establish a routine, that late night out should be an *exception* to the rule, not the rule.

Being consistent with your sleep schedule on the other hand will reinforce your sleep-wake cycle, so you will sleep better.

Pick an hour at which you intend to fall asleep. Then allow for some time to transition from being fully awake to dozing off into dreamland. And when you wake up in the morning, open the curtains as soon as possible to expose yourself to natural light.

In time, you will notice that you will fall asleep more and more easily and feel more and more recharged in the morning, ready to kick off your day.

Sleep Hacks:

- **Go to Sleep and Get Up at Roughly the Same Time Every Day, Also on Weekends**: mixing up your sleep schedule messes with your body's clock, whereas sticking to it reinforces your sleep-wake cycle.

***

15.4 Create A Bedtime Routine

One of the best ways of improving your overall feeling of being rested and recharged is having a bedtime routine. Our brain loves habits and routines, because they help save energy. As we discussed earlier, 40-45% of everything we do on a daily basis is a habit. It happens automatically.

Having a bedtime routine that is the same every day will send a strong message to your brain that it is time to turn off and go to sleep. This starts with the 'cue', which is the trigger for the routine to start.

What is key is that the behavior is roughly the same, day in day out. This is what turns the behavior into a routine, allowing the brain to go on autopilot and reduce the amount of tossing and turning it would otherwise take to fall asleep.

Going to sleep at night and waking up in the morning at the same time are the foundation of an effective bedtime routine.

Another key element is practicing calming activities in the hour or so before heading to bed. You don't need to do the same activity every day, as long as the common denominator is relaxation.

Here are a few things you can do to relax your body:

I. Take a Warm Bath: sitting in the warm water will help you unwind, and increase your body temperature. When you then get out of the bath, your body temperature drops, promoting drowsiness.

II. Listen to Calm Music: during the day, our senses are constantly stimulated. Phone notifications, video advertisements in the subway, people wanting to talk to us. Unfortunately, when we want to fall asleep, we cannot just flip the switch and turn off our brain. It needs some time to calm down.

Listening to calming music can really help counter that. So no Metallica, Justin Bieber, or anything else that may be really stimulating. Instead, try calm, melodic pieces of classical music.

Another good option is listening to brainwave entrainment. These are often long pieces of calm music (twenty minutes or longer) that use binaural beats. The purpose is to lower the frequency of your brainwaves in order to induce drowsiness. By listening to a low audio frequency, your brain will start synchronizing. This can be an easy and very effective way to quickly induce sleep.

III. Keep a Gratitude Journal: as human beings, we have a tendency to pay attention to the negative aspects of our lives. Our brain has been wired with this negativity bias after millions of years of evolution. A negativity bias increases our chances of survival. If we mistakenly take the rock to be a lion, we are more likely to live longer than the other way around. This also explains why you can have a startle response when you mistakenly taking a tree branch for a snake.

However, although it increases our chances of survival, the negativity bias does not make us feel happy and relaxed. We need not be victims of our attention. We can purposefully choose to pay attention to more positive aspects of our life.

A great way of doing this is listing three things for which you are grateful, before you go to sleep, and when you wake up. In a way, we create our own reality by the way we perceive things. We often don't realize how many little things went right today. That croissant was just the right mixture of crunchiness and softness, and had so much flavor. You didn't get hit by a car. The sun was out during your lunch walk. By keeping a gratitude journal, you bring awareness to all the little things that you appreciate in life, which increases your happiness, which in turn will make you feel more relaxed.

IV. Get a Massage: having someone massaging your body can be very calming. It is a good example of how body and mind are connected. A massage reduces your cortisol level, which is a stress hormone, and it simultaneously boosts the production of feel good hormones such as dopamine and serotonin. Many people actually become so relaxed deep into it that they fall asleep during a massage.

If you are familiar with the concept of the book 'The 5 Love Languages' by Gary Chapman, getting a massage is especially beneficial for those whose primary love language is physical touch, as it will make them feel safe and loved even more than those with a different primary love language.

V. Practice Relaxation Exercises: if you don't have someone else to give you a backrub, you need not worry. There are a ton of different relaxation exercises you can practice on your own. Before going to bed, experiment with Qi Gong, Tai Chi or gentle yoga. The slow movements and mild stretches will help your body to de-stress and your mind to unwind, making it easier to fall asleep.

VI. Try Progressive Muscle Relaxation: when you are lying in bed, try progressive muscle relaxation. This involves intentionally tensing your muscles first, and then relaxing them. Hold for about five seconds, and then let go. You can tense up and then relax your whole body all at once, or focus on each muscle group separately. In the latter case, work your way up from the feet to the top of your head.

VII. Perform a Body Scan: this is similar to the progressive muscle relaxation. However, instead of tensing and then relaxing your muscles, you use the power of your awareness to help relax your body.

Performing a body scan is done by bringing your attention to a certain body part, feeling it, and then telling it to relax. Or telling it to go to sleep. Try different commands, see what works best for your body. Start with lying down on your back, and feeling your whole body. Do you feel tension anywhere? Then begin the body scan. Start by bringing your attention to your left leg, followed by your right leg. Next, relax your left and right arm. Relax your pelvic area. Then work your way up from your abdominal area all the way to your neck. Bring your attention to your lower back and work your way up to your shoulders. Continue by relaxing your neck, all the muscles in your face and end at the top of your head. Finally, feel your whole body relaxed.

VIII. Breathe deeply: during the day, we often breathe shallowly. This is because we unconsciously hold on to some tension in our abdominal area. Deep relaxation comes from deep breathing, using the full diaphragm. Taking deep breaths stimulates the parasympathetic nervous system, which governs our 'rest and digest' functions.

Breathing deeply is best practiced lying down. Either let your arms rest besides your body, or place your left hand on your heart and your right hand on your belly. Take a deep inhalation, feeling your abdominal area rise. As you exhale, your belly lowers again. Inhale for about five seconds, hold for a second, and then exhale for five seconds. Take at least fifteen to twenty deep breaths.

To help you keep the right rhythm, try using an app like Breath Pacer (IOS) or Paced Breathing (Android).

If you want to learn more about the power of breathing to relax the body, I highly recommend checking out the Wim Hof Method. This is a 10-week video course created by Wim Hof, aka 'The Iceman'. In it, he teaches the methods he used to climb mount Everest wearing only his shorts and shoes, and complete a marathon above arctic circle in Finland, in temperatures close to -4° Fahrenheit (−20° Celsius). The cornerstone practice of his method is deep breathing. And you don't need to aspire to swim in Antarctic waters in order to benefit from the techniques. You can achieve great relaxation benefits from just practicing the breathing techniques in your bedroom.

IX. Meditate: meditation has been directly linked to countless health benefits, including fighting insomnia and improving sleep. Meditation helps calm the mind and bring awareness to our body, two things that are often missing during our busy days.

There are a number of different meditation practices, but the most basic one is one where you focus on your breath. This practice can be done seated or lying. It is similar to the deep breathing exercise we just spoke about, but, instead of altering your breath, in meditation you merely focus on what is. If you breathe shallowly, high up in your chest area, that is perfectly okay. Just bring your attention there. Feel the breath coming in, staying in your system for a bit, and then leaving your body again. After a while, you will probably notice your breathing becoming more deeply, but don't actively change your breath. The primary goal of meditation is to become aware of whatever is happening in your body right now, and accepting it, with empathy and kindness.

X. Use the Power of Visualization: if worrying about the mortgage can make you feel stressed, by the same rationale visualizing calming scenes should make you feel relaxed, right? When you lie in bed, think of something that you love and calms you down.

For example, one day I woke up from a dream in which a baby elephant was cuddling with me, gently slapping me with its tiny trunk, and being all excited. Visualizing that scene again makes me smile and feel happy.

Other times, I visualize floating in space. I find this to be a very powerful visualization, zooming out from the day-to-day hustle. In space, there are no deadlines, no next episode of Game of Thrones, and no arguments. There is just this immense vastness, and stillness. Experiment with different visualizations and see which ones work for you.

These are just a few strategies to inspire you to create a bedtime routine that is conducive to falling asleep more easily. There are many other things you can do, like lighting candles, a tea ritual, or cuddling with your pet. Be creative here!

But avoid anything that can cause excitement, that stimulates your brain and causes stress. Don't play videogames, work on your laptop, check Facebook, or have a heated discussion in the hour preceding bedtime.

Sleep Hacks:

- **Understand the Power of Creating a Bedtime Routine**: your brains loves habit, to save energy. For a behavior to become a routine though, it needs to be repeated day in day out.

- **Stick to a Sleep Schedule**: this is the most important part of a bedtime routine.
- **Practice Calming Activities in the Hour Before Going to Sleep**. These don't need to be the same every evening, as long as they help you unwind. Experiment with taking a warm bath, keeping a gratitude journal, listening to calm music, getting a massage, practicing relaxation exercises, progressive muscle relaxation or a body scan, breathing deeply, meditating or visualizing calming scenes. And there are many more options. Find the ones which work best for you. But make sure you don't pick anything that stimulates your brain, as this will have the opposite effect.

***

15.5 Keep A Sleep Journal

Keeping track of your daytime activities, the food and drinks you consume, and the times at which you go to bed and wake up, can be really insightful in learning where you can make changes to improve the quality of your sleep.

Sometimes you just cannot see the forest for the trees, but when you track these things and then review your findings later on, you may all of a sudden spot a pattern that is detrimental to sleeping well.

To help you gain insight in your habits, and understand them, keep a journal and track them for two to three weeks. You can buy a variety of sleep journals on sites like Amazon, use the Sleep Diary (goo.gl/8PV614) published by the National Sleep Foundation, or you can opt to use a simple notebook.

Just make sure that, for every day, you track the following:

- What time you went to sleep
- What time you woke up
- What you did in the hour before going to sleep
- How many times you woke up during the night
- A score between 1 - 10 rating the quality of your sleep, where 1 stands for 'horrible' and 10 stands for 'better than Sleeping Beauty'
- A score between 1 - 10 rating how stressful your day was, 1 stands for 'super relaxed' and 10 stands for 'the entire world as I knew it has fallen apart'

- Daily activities, including exercise
- How much coffee and other stimulants you consumed
- Anything else that seems like it could be relevant

After a few weeks, review all your notes and try to see if you can see a pattern, or a causal link. Did you consume coffee excessively on days with low rated sleep quality? Or were you not able to fall asleep on days where you did a vigorous workout?

Keeping track of what you eat and do can help you realize what keeps you awake, and what makes you sleep better. These are clues to how you improve your sleep. Try to implement changes based on your findings, and then keep track of whether these changes indeed cause you to sleep better.

Sleep Hacks:

- **Keep a Sleep Journal**: for two to three weeks, track how and when you sleep, your daytime activities, and what you consume.
- **Review Your Findings**: after those weeks, review your findings and see if you can spot any habits that either keep you awake, or make you sleep better.
- **Test Your Findings**: based on your review, make a few changes to your daily routine, such as reducing your coffee intake. And then track the quality of your sleep again, testing whether assumptions indeed positively impact the quality of your sleep.

***

15.6 Don't Stay In Bed When You Can't Sleep

Have you ever had one of those nights where, no matter what you do or try, you can't fall asleep? Visualizing floating in space, relaxing your body with a body scan, nothing works...

If this happens, don't panic. Going to sleep is not a battle. Trying super hard to fall asleep, and getting upset when it does not happen, is not conducive for dozing off. It is a vicious cycle: your frustration increases your stress, making it even harder to sleep.

If you are widely awake, just tossing and turning, for more than twenty minutes, the best thing you can do is just give in and accept what's in the moment. Get out of bed and wait for sleep to come. Keep the lights turned off, or dimmed at least.

Try one of the relaxing strategies we discussed earlier in this book that you can do outside of your bed, such as mild yoga or meditation. Go back to bed when you start to feel really tired.

And if sleep does not come, picture the worst-case scenario: you won't be able to sleep at all this night, or only for a few hours. That is not the end of the world. There will be many sleep-filled nights in the near future.

Sleep Hacks:

- **If You Are Tossing and Turning For More Than Twenty Minutes, Get Out of Bed**: remember that falling asleep is not a battle. Getting out of bed and waiting to get tired is more conducive to dozing off then building up frustration while lying in bed.
- **When You Are Out of Bed, Engage in a Relaxing Activity**: don't turn on the light, or open Facebook on your phone. Instead, try meditation or another activity that doesn't stimulate your brain.
- **Go Back to Bed When You Feel Tired**: after a while, the urge to go back to bed will come. And if it doesn't, remind yourself that there will be plentiful sleep-filled nights in the near future.

***

15.7 Limit Your Naps

It is tempting to take a nap during the day, especially if you haven't slept that well last night. However, taking long daytime naps can interfere with nighttime sleep.

Therefore, it is best to eliminate naps all together. This way, you will build up the necessary hunger for sleep during the day, which will make you fall asleep more easily come nightfall.

If you feel the urge to take a nap, first try to boost your energy level by drinking a lot of water, striking up a conversation with someone, or getting some fresh air by taking a walk outside.

But if you are sleep deprived, taking a power nap can actually be very beneficial. Studies have shown that a power nap can recharge you, giving you a burst of alertness and increased motor performance. The key thing to keep in mind is that you have got to keep it short, about twenty minutes or so. One study found for example that while napping for up to thirty minutes can improve brain performance, longer naps can have a negative effect on one's performance and sleep quality. When you sleep longer than thirty minutes or so, your body will enter the deep sleep stage. It will be more difficult to wake up from this stage, and you will likely feel groggy when you do.

Also, don't snooze too close to bedtime. The earlier you take the nap, the better. Sleeping during the day can confuse your internal body clock. So if you take a long nap at the end of the afternoon, you will likely pay the price at nighttime. And then you will feel the urge for another long nap the next day...

Sleep Hacks:

- **Avoid Naps if You Have Trouble Falling Asleep at Nighttime**: if you feel the urge to take a nap, drink some water, take a walk or strike up a conversation in order to boost your energy level.
- **Keep Your Naps Short**: taking naps can increase your alertness and overall brain performance, especially if you are sleep deprived. But keep them short, no more

than thirty minutes. Taking longer naps can leave you feeling even more tired.

- **Nap Early**: daytime naps can interfere with nighttime sleep, especially if you take them later in the day. Take your naps in the early afternoon, so that you have enough time to build up enough hunger for sleep before nighttime.

***

15.8 Keep A To-Do List

Do you recognize this? You are lying in bed, ready to nod off, when all of a sudden you have an insight in a problem you have been working on a few days ago. Just a few minutes later, you realize that you need to buy new dog food tomorrow. And, oh wait, you must also not forget to give your daughter money to pay for the upcoming school trip. How are you going to remember all of this?

That's simple: write them down.

As David Allen, the author of the classic productivity book 'Getting Things Done', says: *"Your mind is for having ideas, not holding them."*

Although there are numerous memory training methods out there, generally speaking an untrained mind is terrible at remembering things. Trying to remember all these things not only does not work, but also takes up a lot of headspace. By jotting down whatever comes up, you unclutter your mind, allowing for more clarity during the day and stillness when lying in bed.

Before you go to bed, take out a pen and a piece of paper and write down everything that comes to mind. Don't limit yourself to tasks. Remember a funny quote? Write it down. Or that stunning viewpoint in Malaysia that you once saw in a documentary on National Geographic and hope to visit at some point? Add it to the list. Write down anything that comes to mind!

The purpose is to get everything that comes up in your head onto that piece of paper. Do not censor yourself. When you do this exercise for the first time, you will probably find that more and more things will come up as you write things down. Like you have opened Pandora's box! This is excellent, get it all out there. Review the list in the morning, so you can take action on any tasks that can be done that day.

If you want to take it one step further, take some more time and write about your experiences of the day, at work, or with your partner. And express how they made you feel. By penning down your worries, you get them out of your system, allowing you to drift off more smoothly. Some people even choose to burn the paper on which they wrote down their feelings, as a statement to their unconscious mind that these have now been processed and need not take up any more energy.

Sleep Hacks:

- **Keep a To-Do List in Order to Clear Your Mind**: our brain is not meant to hold on to ideas, but only for having them. Writing your ideas down frees up headspace, making it easier to fall asleep because you don't have to worry about forgetting something.
- **Review Your To Do List in the Morning**: if there are any actionable tasks on the list, perform them, on the same day if possible. Performing a task and checking it off your list will give you a sense of accomplishment, making you feel good about yourself, which is conducive to better sleep.

***

15.9 Use Sleep-Inducing Scents

Another tool you can experiment with to make your bedroom a calm environment are relaxing scents. There are certain smells that can make you sleep more soundly. Especially the scent of lavender has been shown to shorten the ride to sleep town.

For example, lavender has been shown to decrease blood pressure and heart rate, putting the subjects in a more relaxed state. And a small 2005 study found that a sniff of lavender before going to bed resulted in more deep sleep.

Experiment with different scents to find the one that works best for you. Besides lavender, scents like chamomile, rose and sandalwood have also been reported to help induce sleep.

Have a bath with scented oils. Light scented candles, sprinkle a whiff of oil on your pillow or blankets, or simply dab it on your wrists. As an alternative, use a sachet under your pillow, or try reed diffusers or room sprays.

Sleep Hacks:

- **Use a Scent to Help Induce Sleep**: certain scents, such as lavender, have a relaxing effect, inducing sleep and helping you to sleep more soundly.
- **Experiment With Different Scents, to Find the One That Works Best For You**: use different scented oils, candles or room sprays and keep track of which one relaxes you the most. Just because a particular scent works well for others doesn't necessarily mean that it is the one that puts you to sleep most effectively.

***

15.10 Get Checked For Sleep Apnea If You Snore

Snoring is a common problem: according to the National Sleep Foundation, 37 million American adults snore on a regular basis. And although men are at higher risk to snore than women, and snoring becomes more common with age and gaining weight, it affects both genders and all ages.

If you are a loud snorer, you may not only keep your partner awake, but even wake yourself up at times. All the nightly vibrations can leave you with a painful throat in the morning.

And snorers often report feeling sleepy during the day, because their sleep wasn't very restful.

To combat snoring, avoid sleeping on your back. By sleeping on your side, your tongue cannot block the airway. Also avoid drinking alcohol. And if you are overweight, losing some of those pounds can reduce snoring too. One study even found that singing for twenty minutes a day significantly reduced snoring! So sing along with your favorite tunes during your commute, or when you are cooking. You will sleep better, and will have a lot more fun during the day too!

Snoring is not just noisy breathing during sleep. It can also be a sign of sleep apnea, which is a sleep disorder in which your breathing is interrupted and inconsistent. This sleep condition is potentially harmful. Paused breathing during sleep could occur thirty times or more per hour in some people!

To rule out sleep apnea, visit a sleep specialist, a doctor who treats people with sleep problems. To assess whether you have sleep apnea, you will likely have to do a polysomnogram sleep study at a sleep center. This basically means you spend one night sleeping under medical supervision, with sensors attached to your chest, limbs, and other parts of your body. Among other things, these measure your brain activity, blood pressure and eye heart rate.

If you are diagnosed with sleep apnea, the sleep specialist may recommend a custom-made retainer mouthpiece or, if your sleep apnea is more severe, a so-called Continuous Positive Airway Pressure (CPAP) machine. This machine, which is connected to your mouth with a hose and a mask or nose-piece, uses mild air pressure to keep your airway open while you sleep. While it is not the most comfortable way to fall asleep, it can greatly improve the quality of your sleep.

Sleep Hacks:

- **Combat Snoring by Sleeping on Your Side**: By sleeping on your side, your airway won't be blocked by your tongue. Avoiding alcohol, losing weight and singing can also help reduce snoring.
- **Visit a Sleep Specialist to Get Checked For Sleep Apnea**: a sleep apnea is a potentially harmful disorder in which your breathing is interrupted and inconsistent. It is often treated with either wearing a mouthpiece, for mild sleep apnea, or a CPAP machine if the disorder is more severe.

***

15.11 Have Sex Or Masturbate

Most of this book is about keeping your bedroom a sacred place for relaxation. But if you remember, in Chapter 11 we spoke about keeping it for sleep and sex only. Not just sleep...

There are many health benefits to having sex, and reaching the big 'O'. Making love doesn't only make you more sleepy because of the exercise you get, but it also causes the body to release a number of stress-reducing hormones such as oxy-tocin, norepinephrine, serotonin and prolactin.

And you are not out of luck if you don't have a partner: tak-ing the solo train building up to an orgasm can also help you fall asleep more easily. It may be a sleep myth that masturba-tion helps you sleep better. But it may help you fall asleep more easily. One study from the year 2000 found that out of a group of 1,866 American female participants, 32% reported to have masturbated in the previous three months to help go to sleep.

Sleep Hacks:

- **Have Sex or Masturbate Before Going to Sleep**: reaching the big 'O' causes your brain to flood your body with a variety of hormones that reduce stress, improve mood and make you feel relax. You'll sleep like a baby!

***

15.12 Don't Be Afraid To Ask For Help

When you have applied all the sleep hacks in this book, and still find that you are not sleeping well, I recommend seeking professional help.

Perhaps you feel the weight of the world resting on your shoulders, and discussing it with a psychologist could help alleviate some of that.

Your insomnia could also be related to a physical health problem. Besides sleep apnea, there are a variety of disorders or diseases that can cause you to not sleep well, such as:

- restless leg syndrome
- depression
- asthma
- hormone imbalances

See your doctor to rule out any health problems, or get proper treatment. There is no shame in admitting you cannot do everything on your own.

Sleep Hacks:

- **Consult a Doctor or Psychologist if The Quality of Your Sleep Doesn't Improve**: ask for help when you cannot find the solution yourself. There is only so much you can see and do on your own. Don't be too proud or embarrassed to seek professional advice.

PART C

RECAP

16. KEY TAKEAWAYS

There you have it: the keys to the castle!

You now know what sleep is and how it works. And more importantly, you learned a bunch of excellent sleep hacks that will help you fall asleep more easily, sleep deeply, and wake up rested and recharged.

Let's recap all the **Key Takeaways** from **'Part A – Sleep Explained'**:

2. WHAT IS SLEEP

Sleep is a natural and recurring period of rest for the mind and body. During sleep, you are not conscious, you are mostly immobile, and your sensitivity to external stimuli is diminished.

***

3. WHY DO WE SLEEP

There is no definitive answer as to why we sleep. What we do know is that sleep helps conserve energy, repair and rejuvenate the body, and develop the brain. There are many health benefits to getting enough sleep, whereas being sleep deprived can put you at risk for heart disease or a stroke, lower sex drive, and affect your mood.

***

4. HOW DOES SLEEP WORK

Sleep proceeds in 90-minute cycles of NREM and REM sleep. These are not identical: as the night progresses, we spend more time in REM sleep in later sleep cycles. Moreover, the amount of NREM and REM sleep is influenced by the time of day.

***

5. HOW LIGHT AFFECTS YOUR SLEEP

Your circadian rhythm is a body clock that controls when you are alert and sleepy. It is not only influenced by natural factors, but also by external factors such as light, time and melatonin. To improve your sleep quality, make sure you see lots of natural (sun)light during the day, and reduce your light exposure in the evening.

***

6. HOW MUCH SLEEP DO WE NEED

Most people need around seven to eight hours of sleep. Short sleepers can be categorized in two types: natural and habitual short sleepers. Natural short sleepers are rare, but due to a gene mutation they reap the benefits of a full night of sleep in nearly half the time. Habitual short sleepers on the other hand have trained themselves to sleep less. However, they take a risk, as they are not immune to the long-term risks of keeping themselves awake.

***

7. WHY DO WE DREAM

Dreams have fascinated mankind for thousands of years. We now know that dreams mainly occur in REM sleep, are necessary, and being deprived of REM sleep causes all kinds of behavioral changes. Different theories suggest that dreams help us form memories, help our brain to process challenging experiences and emotions, and helps us with our survival. But these are only theories: why we dream still remains very much a mystery.

***

8. WHAT ARE SLEEP DISORDERS

Being sleep deprived can have a detrimental impact on your life. Sleep disorders come in different forms, and the cause can vary depending on the type and severity of the sleep disorder, as well as the individual. Sleep disorders are treated with either medical treatment or psychotherapeutic/behavioral treatment. For the first, consult your physician. The second part of this book contains behavioral strategies you can use to tackle sleep deprivation and improve the quality of your sleep.

17. SLEEP HACKS

Understanding these key takeaways is really helpful. Knowing how sleep works can help you make informed decisions on what patterns and habits you need to change to improve the quality of your sleep.

Knowledge alone won't make you sleep better though. That is why 'Part B – How To Sleep Better' really contains the meat and potatoes of this book. In Chapter 9, We first debunked seven sleep myths, to make sure you won't focus on the wrong things.

When we got that out of the way, you learned a ton of strategies that you can use to hack your sleep.

But real change comes from taking action.

Therefore, let's recap all the **Sleep Hacks** included in '**Part B – How To Sleep Better**':

10. MAKE YOUR BEDROOM A SLEEP SANCTUARY

1. Review Your Bedroom Behaviors: do you reserve your bedroom for sleep and sex only? Or are you playing video games, or working on your laptop?

2. Understand How Habits Work: Be honest with yourself. You may think that what you do in the bedroom besides sleeping isn't really important. But that may simply be a matter of habit. Understand the power of signaling to your brain that you are going to sleep the moment you enter the bedroom.

3. Review Your Bedroom Habits: Use the Cue/Routine/Reward loop to analyze your bedroom habits.

4. Change Your Bedroom Habits: If you spot a bedroom habit that isn't conducive to having a good night sleep, work on changing that habit. Keep in mind though that it takes time to change a habit, or even build a new one. They don't appear overnight. Be patient and compassionate with yourself if you fall back in an old habit. There is always a new day. Success is simply a matter of standing up one more time than you fall.

5. Do The Grandma Test: walk into your room, imagining you are your grandma. Would she be impressed by how calm and clean your room is? Or would she feel the immediate urge to take out a mop and start cleaning it?

6. Ask Yourself: Does Entering Your Bedroom Make You Feel Relaxed?: sometimes we cannot see the forest for trees anymore, because our bedroom is, well...that room where we spend one-third of every day, week in, week out. But if you are having trouble falling asleep, improving the calmness and cleanliness of your bedroom can have a great impact.

7. Keep Your Bedroom Organized: store your clothes in a closet. Store other items under your bed.

8. Keep Your Bedroom Clean: try to clean your bedroom at least once a week.

9. Turn Your Bedroom Into a Calm Environment: paint your walls in a tranquil color. And put up relaxing decorations on the wall.

10. Ventilate Your Bedroom Daily: ideally, sleep with an open window. If that is not possible, open the window during the day. Also consider installing a humidifier or a fan.

11. Don't Be a Perfectionist: apply the 20/80 rule, where you identify the 20% of the changes that will have 80% of the desired result of having a clean bedroom that calms the mind when you enter it.

12. Check Your Bedroom Temperature: what is the temperature in your bedroom when you go to sleep? And how do you feel when you are in bed: just right, or do you regularly feel too warm or too cold?

13. Test Which Bedroom Temperature is Most Comfortable For You: for one week, keep a sleep journal. Score the quality of your sleep, while experimenting with different room temperatures.

14. Set Your Ideal Bedroom Temperature: depending on your test results, adjust the room temperature to your liking. Be creative: consider installing an air conditioner, if you don't have one. Or keep the window open at night to ventilate the room. Alternatively, if your room is too cold, wear some pajamas and/or put an extra blanket on your bed.

15. Live in a Quiet Neighborhood: don't live next to a nightclub in the middle of the city if you are a light sleeper.

16. Make Sure Your Bedroom is as Far Away as Possible From the External Noise: make sure your bedroom is in the back of the house, if the front side of your house is on a busy road.

17. Improve the Isolation of Your Bedroom Walls and Windows: isolating your bedroom walls can make a great difference in keeping out distracting sounds. The same goes for double or triple glazing.

18. Turn on a Fan or a White Noise Machine: the whir or a fan or white noise machine is not only soothing, but also reduces the impact of disruptive noises.

19. Wear Earplugs: even the simplest foam earplugs can greatly improve the quality of your sleep. If you have some more money to spend, consider buying noise-masking earplugs.

20. Make Your Bedroom as Dark as Possible: turn off all lights, and use dark curtains or blackout shades.

21. Try Wearing a Sleep Mask: though some people find wearing a sleep mask uncomfortable, it is great tool to block out any light.

***

11. TURN YOUR BED INTO A SLEEP HAVEN

22. Sleep On a Comfortable Mattress: there is no such thing as a 'one size fits all mattress'. A good mattress for you is the one on which YOU feel no pressure. It supports your body in a neutral position.

23. Check In On How You Feel When You Wake Up: how do you feel when you wake up in the morning? If you often experience back pain in the morning, this may be an indication that it is time to replace your mattress.

24. Replace Your Mattress After Seven To Ten Years: a mattress does not have eternal life. If you have slept on your mattress for years, start looking for a new mattress, especially if you wake up with physical discomforts.

25. Try Before You Buy: when buying a new mattress, take the time to test it. Comfort is more important than price. Which mattress you buy is going to impact the quality of your sleep for years to come, so you do not want to make this decision lightly. If you do not test the mattress, you might regret it later.

26. Sleep Under a Warm Blanket: the number and thickness of the blankets depends on the season. Make sure you are warm enough, but don't overheat.

27. Rest Your Head on a Comfortable Pillow: which one is best depends on your body, sleeping position, and personal preference. Test before you buy.

28. Use Just One Pillow: piling up pillows can cause tension on your neck and spine. Just use one pillow that comfortable supports your head and neck.

29. Use a Pillow to Support Other Parts of Your Body: sleeping with a pillow between your legs, or under your knees can help alleviate tension in your hips or lower back

30. Replace Your Pillow at Least Every Two Years: a pillow that is past its due date can do more damage than good.

31. Limit Your Bed Activities to Sleep and Sex Only: by doing so, you send a strong signal to your brain that your bed is a sacred space for relaxation only.

32. Ask Yourself if Your Pet Cuts Your Sleep Short: sure, you love falling asleep with your furry friend besides you. But does your dog or cat regularly wake you up in the middle of the night?

33. If So, Keep Your Pet Out of The Bedroom: this may take some time to get used to, both for you and your pet. Don't give in to the temptation to bring your pet back in the bedroom. Improving the quality of your sleep is the most important, and you will both get used to the new situation eventually. Plus, a little time apart has never hurt a relationship. You and your pet will be super excited to see each other the next morning!

34. Consult an Animal Trainer or Vet: if your pet is having a lot of trouble adjusting to the new situation, considering asking your animal trainer or vet to help your pet transition to sleeping happily elsewhere in the house.

35. If You Have Allergy Symptoms, Keep Your Pet Out and Clean Your Bedroom: pets carry around allergy triggers like fleas or pollen. Also, accumulated dust can affect your respiratory system.

36. If the Symptoms Remain, Take an Allergy Test: within minutes after taking it, a skin prick test will show you if you have any type of allergy.

37. Vigorously Clean Up Your Room if You Have a Dust Mite Allergy: dust mites feed of skin flakes. A good place to start is replacing your bedding, and encase it with dust mite covers. Also replace your carpet for a hard floor. After that, it is a matter of keeping your room clean. Clean your bedding at least once a week with hot water, and your floor with a HEPA vacuum cleaner.

38. Make Your Bed Every Morning: this will improve the quality of your sleep. It will also be your first completed task, kick starting a productive day. And if your day didn't go as planned, at least you can come home to nicely made bed, and start anew tomorrow.

39. If Your Partner is a Bed Hog, Try Separate Sheets and Duvets: you can still cuddle before falling asleep, but when you go to sleep it is less likely that your partner's movements will wake you up.

40. If Your Partner Snores, Try Earplugs First, and Otherwise Visit a Physician: snoring can be an indication of sleep apnea, so it is a good idea to have a physician take a look at it and recommend what steps to take. If nothing helps, sleeping in another room might be your last option.

41. Whatever Sleep Position You Are in, Set the Intention to Keep Your Head and Neck Straight: this will improve the quality of your sleep.

42. Try Sleeping Naked: numerous studies have shown the health benefits of sleeping naked, such as sleeping more deeply and reducing stress.

***

12. GET YOUR LIGHT FIX DURING THE DAY, DIM THE LIGHTS AT NIGHT

43. Dim the Lights: dim the lights in the evening, or change a few light bulbs to a lower wattage.

44. Eliminate All Sources of Light in Your Bedroom: remove or cover any sources of artificial light in your bedroom.

45. Experiment With Natural Light: light candles or a fire.

46. Expose Yourself to Daylight as Soon as You Wake Up: bright daylight sends a strong message to your brain that it is time to wake up.

47. Have a Break? Go Outside: whenever you have time during the day, take that opportunity to go outside. These little bits of daylight exposure add up over the day and keep your circadian rhythm healthy.

***

13. STAY AWAY FROM ELECTRONIC DEVICES IN THE EVENING

48. Establish an Electronic Curfew: one hour before you go to sleep, turn off your television, phone, laptop, and any other electrical devices.

49. Limit Your Exposure To Blue Light: turn off your electronic devices a couple of hours before you go to bed, and keep them another room.

50. If This Is Too Hardcore, At Least Install F.lux or a Similar Color Filter App to Reduce Your Exposure To Blue Light: the filtered colors are easier on the eyes, making it easier to fall asleep later. keep your electronics in another room, use a color filter app, or reduce the brightness. You can also reduce the brightness on your device.

51. Don't Hop on Phone Calls an Hour Before Going to Sleep: doing calls just before bedtime may negatively influence the production of melatonin, and also doesn't help in calming your mind.

52. Set Your Phone Mute To Silent Mode: if you can't get yourself to turn off your electronic devices, at least turn your phone on mute, to prevent getting distracted or woken up.

***

14. CHANGE YOUR DIET

53. Avoid Eating Heavy Meals in the Evening: your body is meant to recharge during sleep, not digest food.

54. Don't Eat Anything Two Hours Before Going to Sleep: don't go to bed hungry. But by making sure you consume enough calories during the day, you won't need to eat anything in the hours preceding sleep, and it will make falling asleep easier.

55. Include Foods in Your Diet That Are Rich in Magnesium and Tryptophan: these can be found in foods like turkey, green leafy vegetables and bananas. Eating these foods during the day will help induce sleep at night.

56. Drink Two Liters of Water Every Day: drinking enough water energizes your entire system, and lets you sleep deeper.

57. Don't Drink Any Liquids Two Hours Before Going to Sleep: drinking liquids before bedtime can result in waking up to urinate. If your mouth runs dry late at night, sip on a cup of herbal tea. And go to the bathroom before heading to bed.

58. Don't Consume Caffeine After 2 p.m.: caffeine is a stimulant that can stay in your system for six to eight hours. It is fine to drink coffee in the morning. But don't consume any caffeine later in the day, so your Zzzs are not affected.

59. Don't Drink Alcohol Before Going to Sleep: you may fall asleep more easily, but it comes at a cost: alcohol interferes with your sleep by reducing REM sleep, leaving you feeling less rested and recharged in the morning.

60. Quit Smoking: nicotine is a stimulant that can keep you awake and leave you feeling unrested in the morning.

15. OTHER STRATEGIES TO IMPROVE SLEEP QUALITY

61. Exercise Daily: you don't need to perform at the level of an Olympic athlete in order to improve the quality of your sleep. What is most important is having a routine where you exercise regularly, ideally every day. Acknowledge the level where you are at now, and start building your fitness from there.

62. Don't Do Vigorous Exercise Within Four Hours of Going to Bed: although you may be the exception to the rule, most people will feel very energetic and awake in the first hours after finishing their workout. Therefore, it is best to not do any strong exercise shortly before going to bed.

63. Practice Gentle Exercises That Bring About Relaxation Instead: exercises like Qi Gong, Tai Chi or gentle yoga connect mind and body and will help you to feel more relaxed. Check out my book 'Yoga For Beginners: 10 Super Easy Poses To Reduce Stress and Anxiety' to learn ten easy beginner techniques that will help release stress and anxiety, making you feel more relaxed and fall asleep more easily. You can access it here: amazon.com/dp/B01N4ATAQY.

64. Go to Sleep and Get Up at Roughly the Same Time Every Day, Also on Weekends: mixing up your sleep schedule messes with your body's clock, whereas sticking to it reinforces your sleep-wake cycle.

65. Understand the Power of Creating a Bedtime Routine: your brains loves habit, to save energy. For a behavior to become a routine though, it needs to be repeated day in day out.

66. Stick to a Sleep Schedule: this is the most important part of a bedtime routine.

67. Practice Calming Activities in the Hour Before Going to Sleep. These don't need to be the same every evening, as long as they help you unwind. Experiment with taking a warm bath, keeping a gratitude journal, listening to calm music, getting a massage, practicing relaxation exercises, progressive muscle relaxation or a body scan, breathing deeply, meditating or visualizing calming scenes. And there are many more options. Find the ones which work best for you. But make sure you don't pick anything that stimulates your brain, as this will have the opposite effect.

68. Keep a Sleep Journal: for two to three weeks, track how and when you sleep, your daytime activities, and what you consume.

69. Review Your Findings: after those weeks, review your findings and see if you can spot any habits that either keep you awake, or make you sleep better.

70. Test Your Findings: based on your review, make a few changes to your daily routine, such as reducing your coffee intake. And then track the quality of your sleep again, testing whether assumptions indeed positively impact the quality of your sleep.

71. If You Are Tossing and Turning For More Than Twenty Minutes, Get Out of Bed: remember that falling asleep is not a battle. Getting out of bed and waiting to get tired is more conducive to dozing off then building up frustration while lying in bed.

72. When You Are Out of Bed, Engage in a Relaxing Activity: don't turn on the light, or open Facebook on your phone. Instead, try meditation or another activity that doesn't stimulate your brain.

73. Go Back to Bed When You Feel Tired: after a while, the urge to go back to bed will come. And if it doesn't, remind yourself that there will be plentiful sleep-filled nights in the near future.

74. Avoid Naps if You Have Trouble Falling Asleep at Nighttime: if you feel the urge to take a nap, drink some water, take a walk or strike up a conversation in order to boost your energy level.

75. Keep Your Naps Short: taking naps can increase your alertness and overall brain performance, especially if you are sleep deprived. But keep them short, no more than thirty minutes. Taking longer naps can leave you feeling even more tired.

76. Nap Early: daytime naps can interfere with nighttime sleep, especially if you take them later in the day. Take your naps in the early afternoon, so that you have enough time to build up enough hunger for sleep before nighttime.

77. Keep a To-Do List in Order to Clear Your Mind: our brain is not meant to hold on to ideas, but only for having them. Writing your ideas down frees up headspace, making it more easy to fall asleep because you don't have to worry about forgetting something.

78. Review Your To Do List in the Morning: if there are any actionable tasks on the list, perform them, on the same day if possible. Performing a task and checking it off your list will give you a sense of accomplishment, making you feel good about yourself, which is conducive to better sleep.

79. Use a Scent to Help Induce Sleep: certain scents, such as lavender, have a relaxing effect, inducing sleep and helping you to sleep more soundly.

80. Experiment With Different Scents, to Find the One That Works Best For You: use different scented oils, candles or room sprays and keep track of which one relaxes you the most. Just because a particular scent works well for others doesn't necessarily mean that it is the one that puts you to sleep most effectively.

81. Combat Snoring by Sleeping on Your Side: By sleeping on your side, your airway won't be blocked by your tongue. Avoiding alcohol, losing weight and singing can also help reduce snoring.

82. Visit a Sleep Specialist to Get Checked For Sleep Apnea: a sleep apnea is a potentially harmful disorder in which your breathing is interrupted and inconsistent. It is often treated with either wearing a mouthpiece, for mild sleep apnea, or a CPAP machine if the disorder is more severe.

83. Have Sex or Masturbate Before Going to Sleep: reaching the big 'O' causes your brain to flood your body with a variety of hormones that reduce stress, improve mood and make you feel relax. You'll sleep like a baby!

84. Consult a Doctor or Psychologist if The Quality of Your Sleep Doesn't Improve: ask for help when you cannot find the solution yourself. There is only so much you can see and do on your own. Don't be too proud or embarrassed to seek professional advice.

***

We started this book with the following quote by the pioneering sleep researcher William Dement:

"You're not healthy, unless your sleep is healthy"

By applying these sleep hacks, you will be able to take back control of your life again. And after a healthy night's rest where you slept like a baby, you will wake up full of energy, ready to jumpstart your day!

18. ONE LAST THING...

Thank you for picking up a copy of this book, and sticking around all the way to the end. I'm impressed: this tells me you have the willpower to push through in difficult times, and you will be able make permanent changes in your life. I really hope that everything you learned in this book will help you improve the quality of your sleep!

If you enjoyed this book or found it useful, I would like to ask you for a favor. Would you be kind enough to share your thoughts and post a review of this book on Amazon? You can search for it on Amazon, or go to:

bit.ly/insomniareview

Your support really does make a difference. It helps bring it under the attention of other people who may also suffer from sleep deprivation and could benefit from the strategies laid out in this book. And I read all the reviews personally, so I can get your feedback and use that to make this book even better.

Thank you again for buying this book and I wish you will sleep even better than Disney's Sleeping Beauty! Just make sure you wake up again. Seriously. Life is so much fun after a good night sleep!

ALSO BY THE SAME AUTHOR

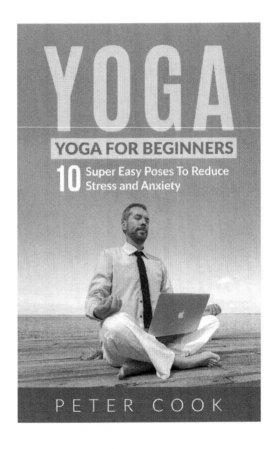

Read it here:
bit.ly/cookyogabeginner

☆☆Download Today! 10 Super Easy Yoga Poses Yoga To End Your Stress And Feel Happy Again! ☆☆

Ask yourself:

- Do you worry a lot?

- Are you having trouble falling asleep?

- Have you recently snapped at someone over something small, like not doing the dishes?

Did you answer one or more of these questions with **yes?** Then it is likely that you have been under **too much stress** for too long.

I have good news for you though: You can take back control of your life.

I should know.

I have personally experimented with many different techniques to reduce stress. And yoga is unique in that it combines physical exercise with a mental awareness. And this is crucial if you want to reduce stress.

I was so inspired that I wanted to learn everything I could about how it works: I have **almost 1,000 hours of different Yoga Teacher Trainings** under my belt. I learned how yoga and meditation can calm the mind and body, AND end stress and anxiety like no other form of exercises. Now I want to share my experience and the knowledge I have gained with you. So I can help you improve the quality of life!

Dr. Dean Ornish said it wonderfully in the documentary 'Yoga Unveiled':

"Yoga doesn't bring you a sense of peace, health or well-being. It's not like taking valium. Rather, it helps you quiet down your mind and body. So you can experience what your true nature is, which is to be peaceful until we disturb it."

Take back control of your life and happiness: start learning how you can end stress and anxiety for good with these easy yoga poses anyone can do!

Here's what I want you to do:

Read this book. Practice the yoga poses. And end your stress!

Here Is A Preview Of What You Will Learn...

- Ten Simple And Easy Yoga Poses to Eliminate Stress and Anxiety

- What Stress Is

- Why Your Perception of Stress is so Important

- What Yoga Really is

- How Doing Yoga Can Reduce Stress

- That Yoga is For EVERYBODY: Men, Women, Kids. All Can Benefit!

- Why Yoga Differs From Other Types of Exercise in Reducing Stress and Anxiety

- How to Meditate

- And Much More Valuable Content!

Here is what other readers have said about *'Yoga For Beginners: 10 Super Easy Poses To Reduce Stress and Anxiety'*:

"I totally recommend this book.

I bought the paper version and I am very satisfied with my purchase.

The book is really well organised and easy to follow. You would not get bored or lost. The content is perfectly adapted to beginners like me.

It starts with a very personal introduction that in my case was very helpful to keep my interest alive. I saw myself in the personal experience of the author and how yoga has helped him dealing with stress.

The yoga poses are super easy to follow and the fact of having pictures makes it even easier.

Great resource for starting out with yoga or if you are simply looking for a solution on how to understand and control your stress."

Susana Nakatani

"This is a perfect introduction to some of the most practical and useful tools to reduce stress and anxiety. I have tried a bunch of different yoga classes before, it's hard to find what's valuable in between all the strange words for poses, and to know what specifically works for me. This book gave me a simple and easy routine to do each morning and clearly explains the benefits."

Kyle

"This is a wonderful introduction to yoga and learn how to reduce stress and anxiety. We all are a bit stressed out with all the demands of our daily life and every now and then have to deal with anxiety. Peter Cook does an excellent job to demystify yoga for everybody and gives practical advice on how to deal with stress and anxiety. The explanation of the poses are on point and easy to follow. I gave the book to my male friend who thinks yoga is only for women and even he got interested, good job!"

Monika Werner

So...ARE YOU READY TO TAKE ACTION?

==> ACT NOW!

Go to:

bit.ly/cookyogabeginner

and click the 'buy' button to get your copy today!

"Usually, when people get to the end of a chapter, they close the book and go to sleep. I deliberately write a book so when the reader gets to the end of the chapter, he or she must turn one more page."

Sidney Sheldon

54553546R00102

Made in the USA
Middletown, DE
04 December 2017